The
Evolution
Diet

All-Natural
and
Allergy Free

Joseph Stephen Breese Morse

With Foreword by Holly Petty, Ph.D.

This book was produced by Amelior Publishing Company, an imprint of Code Publishing, San Diego, CA. www.code-interactive.com/amelior

ISBN 1-60020-047-8

978-1-60020-047-2

Contents

Foreword
Holly Petty, Ph.D.

In primitive times, we did not live to eat, but ate to live. So often it is the opposite now, we live to eat and we have strayed from the way, not only how we should eat, but live. Joseph Morse provides us with a way of eating by primordial, tangible examples in *The Evolution Diet: All-Natural and Allergy Free*. Joseph provides a strong historical backdrop, forming a solid foundation, from which the reader can learn and embrace the diet of our ancestors' years ago. In *The Evolution Diet*, Joseph reveals a way of eating to moderation and happiness.

Joseph shared his Evolution Diet with me, and I found it very comparable to the way in which I already ate, fruits and berries by day, little nibbles and bits if you will, and eating meat and vegetables at night. With great excitement and delight, I shared with him that I followed this Evolution Diet because I suffer from various food allergies. Through trial and error, I came upon a consistent way of eating, following an eating plan that leaves me feeling happy and healthy without suffering from allergies.

Joseph reveals that, "The Evolution Diet as a way to work *with* your body, and not against it like so many modern diets do." Indeed, The Evolution Diet was my allergy free solution as I was listening to my body and not adhering to the traditional American food staples. With compassion for the food intolerant and food allergic, Joseph provides a clear introduction to food allergies, what allergens are most common in America (the "Big Eight" allergens (fish, shellfish, milk, egg, soy, wheat, peanuts, and tree nuts) and why primitive man may not have eaten these foods, and how we came to eat these foods today. By writing *The Evolution Diet: All-Natural and Allergy Free*, Joseph opened another door by which food challenged individuals can also follow The Evolution Diet, with special reference to common allergens and to meals that do not contain specific allergens.

With wit, research, and a diet plan, Joseph sets out to rid the reader's mind of diet fallacies. A diet is not a specific way of eating for a predetermined time but for life, and Joseph provides information by which we can eat healthfully and happily.

As with the hunters of long ago, we seek out to satisfy our hunger, perhaps not with a spear, but following Joseph Morse's *The Evolution Diet: All-Natural and Allergy Free*, we can do so with a well-informed, sharp mind.

Thank you Joseph, my friend, for the opportunity to contribute to your book, so that we may help better the lives of the reading consumer through diet, particularly for those who suffer from food allergies.

Part One

The Evolution Diet
(An All-Natural and Allergy Free Life)

"One should eat to live, not live to eat."

- Cicero

It was an important morning for Kashe because he was setting off on his first hunting expedition with four men of the village. Earlier, the 14-year-old Kashe had only played hunting; never had he actually gone on one of the noblest missions for a man. He was envisioning it in his mind how he would be the one to throw the final spear into the hunted beast and slay it for good.

The villagers set off with Kashe early that morning each equipped with a water pouch and a bow complete with five or six hand-made poison-tipped arrows made out of wood and bone and one large spear. They walked directly east, and then picked up the trail of a gemsbok, a large African antelope. The lead tracker, Musaka, could tell that the gemsbok tracks were fresh because of the sharp edges they still maintained in the sandy ground, and after half a day of tracking, they were led to the giant animal enjoying some afternoon shade with his small herd about 20 kilometers from the village.

The hunters targeted the largest gemsbok. It was enormous—nearly 500 pounds, Musaka estimated. The hunters crouched down and slowly and quietly inched within striking distance of the animal. Once they were close enough, they raised their bows all at once and fired on the animal.

Suddenly everything exploded and the herd bolted. The hunters ran after the wounded beast for a couple hundred meters and finally the gemsbok turned back to fight. The hunters approached the large beast and launched their man-made spears at it, but the gemsbok fiercely warded them off with its three-foot-long razor-like antlers. Finally, Musaka got a clean shot and struck the animal in the neck, killing it. The scene calmed down and the hunters began to take stock of what had happened.

Where's Kashe? They all wondered.

"I'm up here," he yelled down from a nearby tree in his native tongue. When the gemsbok had stood its ground, Kashe got scared and leaped into a tree. Musaka laughed, "Ha ha ha. If it was up to you to feed the village, Kashe, we would all starve!" Everyone got a good laugh out of that.

The hunters tied the prey onto wooden rods, supported the enormous beast on their shoulders, and headed back to the village where the women and children were sorting out the days collection of nuts and berries. It was the beginning of the wet season in the area and one of the village's women, Sanni was very pleased with the choices of tasty foods available. On her foraging walk just a few kilometers from her family's camp, Sanni foraged an abundance of green leafy vegetables, tasty berries, and nutritious nuts.

She had gathered more food on that trip than she had in months and was very pleased.

After snacking on nuts, fruits, and vegetables all day, the women butchered the gemsbok, cooked it, and everyone filled themselves on the nutritious meat. At the campfire, Kashe couldn't help but smile as Musaka told of his embarrassing story. "I guess I'm not ready to become a man yet," Kashe explained and everyone laughed.

This story may seem like one about an ancient Stone Age hunter/gatherer society whose only connection to the present is through fossilized bones and burial remains. But the story of Kashe, Musaka, and Sanni takes place today in a region of southwest Africa in the Kalahari Desert where various groups of !Kung Bushmen—nomadic tribes of hunter/gatherers—still exist.

Geneticist Spencer Wells, who has studied the !Kung in depth, reckons that the !Kung family line is the oldest on Earth—a "genetic Adam" from which everyone can trace their ancestral lineage—and that not much has changed for them since their distant relatives left Africa some 50,000 years ago. For instance, the !Kung still maintain their ancient language that incorporates popping and clicking (the exclamation mark before the 'Kung' in their name represents the sound generated by quickly pulling down your tongue). In addition, many of the Bushmen tribes around the area have also maintained a traditional hunter/gatherer lifestyle described above.

In fact, the !Kung are probably the largest group of hunter/gatherers left on Earth, and what is remarkable is that many subsets of the !Kung people live completely without any agriculture or domesticated animals whatsoever. Not only do they persevere in an extremely challenging climate, but they also seem to be doing it in impressive fashion. Over 10 percent of the Bushmen are over

60 years old (16 percent of Americans are beyond that threshold), a stunning figure given the lack of modern medicine. And by most accounts, the Bushmen are a cheerful people. As one !Kung member put it, they do what their hearts want; they are not poor; they have everything they could care about.

It seems the only real threat to the !Kung way of life is the government's forced modernization policy which has relocated many Bushmen into permanent housing settlements, a plan that many have claimed is a way to clear the area for lucrative diamond mining and tourism. When the Bushmen are relocated to settlements and removed from their natural hunter/gatherer lifestyle, the results are tragic, to say the least. For the 1,800 or so Bushmen that were relocated into camps over the past decades, the quality of life has rapidly deteriorated and many have contracted HIV/AIDS, tuberculosis, or become dependent on alcohol.

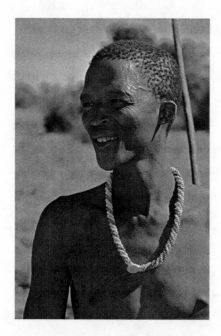

A modern hunter/gatherer !Kung Bushman of the Kalahari

The government insists that they provide drinking water and basic health care at the camps, but the Bushmen of the Kalahari were able to procure enough drinking water in the middle of the desert so as to survive for thousands of years without government help; wasn't that enough? Additionally, basic medical care is good, but only becomes vital when people are forced to live in cramped quarters where disease tends to thrive. As one relocated !Kung woman reported of the camps, "There are too many people; there's no food to gather; game is far away and people are dying of tuberculosis. When I was a little girl,

 An Evolution Diet Essential

Returning to a natural hunter/gatherer diet immediately reduces risk of degenerative diseases like cardiovascular conditions.

we left sickness behind us when we moved." In other words, her childhood hunter/gatherer lifestyle was without a doubt healthier than the government-mandated settlement living. A major component of that lifestyle was the diet.

Most of the scientific literature backs up what that !Kung woman felt for herself intuitively. One study, conducted in Australia, aimed to see if Aborigines who had been assimilated into a Western-style diet could become healthier by returning to their former hunter/gatherer lifestyle. The findings were striking. Seven weeks of the traditional natural diet showed a marked decrease in blood lipid levels and blood glucose levels of the test subjects. In other words, the Western diet had made the Aborigines overweight and gave them increased chance of cardiovascular disease and diabetes. Returning to the natural hunter/gatherer lifestyle fixed all that.

The Evolution Diet aims to bring us all back to that happy and healthy place that Kashe, Musaka, and Sanni lived—full of a joy for food and the health it brings—without leaving the comforts of modern living. By reintroducing into your life the foods and habits of the hunter/gatherer peoples like the present-day !Kung and the ancestors of all mankind, you too can reap the rewards of longevity, ideal weight, and reduced risk of degenerative disease.

What's on the menu?

The !Kung Bushmen (also known as the !Kung San) have adapted to their desert surroundings quite well, keeping close to water and procuring food from a wide variety of plants and animals. Every adult in the typical !Kung clan is involved in foraging and/or hunting. The most important staple in the !Kung San diet is the mongongo nut (what they call the //"xa), which has the macronutrient equivalent of peanuts—high in fat and protein and many vitamins and minerals. The tree also shares a fruit in the summer that has a nutritional composition complementary to the nut (high in carbohydrates and other vitamins and minerals).

Another staple is the baobab fruit, which is rich in vitamin C, calcium, and magnesium. The tsin bean and the vegetable ivory fruit are also attractive options on the !Kung people's Kalahari menu. In all, there are over 100 species of plants that make up the !Kung diet including roots, bulbs, berries, melons, and edible gums. If you don't think 100 species is a lot, I challenge you to write down 100 species of plants that you consume on a regular basis—you may be surprised at what you come up with!

With regard to meat, the !Kung diet is just as diverse. Anything from large game to small animals can be found on the menu. The hunters of the camp (usually men) will go out on a hunting expedition for up to 6 days in search of big antelope, kudu, wildebeest, and gemsbok, armed with poison-tipped arrows. When the hunters return, the village feasts on the fresh meat. In all, meat comprises from 20-50 percent of the !Kung diet by weight. When big game is not available due to the season, smaller mammals (usually trapped by the women of the village) supplement the diet.

So, there you have it, the typical hunter/gatherer diet: nuts, fruits, roots, and berries throughout the day and wild-animal meat after the hunt. It is the definition of healthy eating and is what sustained the human species (the descendants of the !Kung and you) through hundreds of thousands of years. This is the diet what we promote in The Evolution Diet.

When you extend the principles of the !Kung to natural hunter/gatherers in different ages and regions of the world, the menu opens up to an array of similar all-natural and allergy free foods. To start, the !Kung don't fish, but that's certainly due to the lack of fisheries and rivers in the middle of the Kalahari desert, not due to lack of ability or distaste for fish. Most of what we know about ancient hunter/gatherer societies is that fishing was a main component of their existence and if there were any coastal hunter/gatherers around today, we'd probably find the same thing. In fact, the closest to that lifestyle is shared with the Inuit people of the Arctic Circle, who almost exclusively eat fish. The Evolution Diet doesn't just recommend mongongo nuts and fruit; it promotes pretty much all fruits and vegetables and all lean meats.

In this respect, the natural hunter/gatherer diet is diverse. Whereas the typical Western diet derives nearly all of its vegetarian foods from a few staple crops (corn, soybeans, wheat, rice), and most of the meat comes from animals fed with the same four crops (most likely corn), the !Kung and others like them are open to nearly all of nature's bounty.

There are things that typical Westerners eat that traditional hunter/gatherers don't eat, however. Some noticeable foods missing from the above rundown of a natural hunter/gatherer diet are grasses (such as wheat), dairy products (such as milk), and legumes, among others. The main reason that the !Kung Bushmen and other hunter/gatherers avoided these foods is that they are toxic (or at least indigestible) in their raw state, making them what nutritionists have termed anti-nutrients. Uncooked wheat contains phytate, which binds important minerals like magnesium and calcium in our bodies, contributing to mineral deficiencies. Milk contains the sugar lactose, which cannot be digested by a majority of the adult population. And soybeans contain hemagglutinins, which promote red blood cell clumping and significantly suppresses growth.

So, naturally, if prehistoric hunter/gatherers ate those foods, they would not have lasted as long as they did and perhaps our species would have ceased to exist. But something happened about 10,000 years ago — humans discovered cooking. At that time, some brilliant caveman or woman somehow thought to heat up his mush made of grains and water instead of using it as Silly Putty and, voilà, the village had bread! Around the same time, people started to ferment the milk products from their family cows and were able to produce cheese or yogurt. There were, of course, benefits to this cooked form of grain and milk product; they were easier to transport and easy to store; they were dense in calories; and, most importantly, they weren't nearly as toxic as their raw counterparts. Cooking eliminates many of the toxins in grains and milk (and many beans and potatoes for that matter) and opens up mankind to a vast amount of food previously untouchable. For many species of plants, cooking equals eating.

And so, mankind ate and ate the newly available foods. And when it became obvious that the food was also the seed (as is the case in grains and beans), some other smart Neolithic ancestors got the bright idea that if they used some of the food to plant more, they would eventually have a lot more food. This process slowly evolved into farming and some of those foods that were toxic to humans before the concept of cooking took hold eventually became the most popular foods on Earth. Notice that two of these formerly toxic foods (wheat and soybeans) are among the highest consumed plant foods for Westerners today.

But while the super-staple foods derived from wheat and soybeans (along with other indigestible plants and animal byproducts) helped populate the Earth with their dense calories, there are problems with those plants being used as foods. As we will see more clearly in Part Five, cooking eliminates most of the toxins in grains and beans, but not all of them. When we eat those foods, we still take in chemicals that we were not evolved to eat and when we rely on those foods for most of our diet, the results are not good.

The original Evolution Diet allowed for certain amounts of whole-grain wheat, soy, and non-toxic bean foods because they closely match the macronutrient content of other low-sugar, high-fiber (what we'll term LoS Hi-Fi) foods that are integral to the natural hunter/gatherer diet. However, it should be noted that over-reliance on the aforementioned toxic foods can be dangerous. In addition, there is a large portion of the population who cannot eat even a small amount of the foods because of allergies or digestive intolerances. Celiac disease (gluten intolerance), lactose intolerance, peanut allergies, and other conditions arise because we simply weren't designed to eat the types of foods that many Westerners consume daily. That is why *The Evolution Diet: All-Natural and Allergy Free* is necessary. There is no other nutritional plan that specifies exactly what natural hunter/gatherers ate (nuts, berries, vegetables, roots, fish, lean meats, fowl) and in what manner (snacking on LoS Hi-Fi foods throughout the day, then eating a large high-protein meal after exercise). With an overview of human physiology, the cultural and personal aspects that affect our diet, and a detailed look at what and how we were designed to eat, you will be well on your way to living a healthy, all-natural, and allergy free life.

A popular trend from this young 21st century is the concept of detoxification or body cleansing. This process aims at eliminating the caffeine, alcohol, Burger King or other heavily processed foods, trans fats, or some other so-called toxin from one's body by usually just ingesting water, fruits, and vegetables, or special teas (note: there are many other types of detox). While the process has fallen out of favor by the mainstream medical profession, body cleansing has its proponents simply because the feeling to cleanse one's system is so strong with today's unnatural diet and detoxing usually works, on a psychosomatic level as well as a physiological level. Returning to the natural state of diet is a healthy process and The All-Natural and Allergy Free Evolution Diet can be seen almost as a permanent detox. Why stress your system with chemicals and foods that you weren't designed to consume? Why settle with too much weight, bad sleep, or unbalanced energy? Why not evolve into the picture of health that you were meant to be and know you can achieve?

The Evolution Diet

Get to and maintain your ideal weight. Feel healthy and energetic throughout the day. Sleep well every night. These are the goals for many of us today and *The Evolution Die: All-Natural and Allergy Free* is the vehicle that will help us attain them.

If you've ever been curious as to how the human body works or why we eat the things we do, this is the book for you. You are about to embark on an insightful, inspirational journey, as you learn not just what your body is designed to eat, but how and when you should eat it. You'll learn exactly what you're your body is expecting you to feed it and how it will react if you don't do just that. These time-tested principles can't be found in the most advanced scientific or medical technology, though; nor can they be seen in slick marketing gimmicks from multi-million dollar weight loss programs. The principles of ideal health can only be found in our ancestry and in our basic physical makeup.

For nearly two million years, humans and our hominid ancestors were eating in the hunter/gatherer style, much like that of the !Kung from the previous chapters, which consisted of foraging for a wide variety of healthy fruits and vegetables and then hunting and scavenging for large game. Our species was uniquely evolved to eat in this manner based on our place in nature and our ancestors were very successful at it—so successful

 An Evolution Diet Essential

The goal is to imitate the diet of natural humans (those without out strong cultural influences) and to fit the diet for which our bodies have been naturally designed.

that they were able to rocket to the top of the food chain in a matter of generations. However, about 9,000 years ago, most humans started eating in a different way; our species learned how to plant crops for high yields and Homo sapiens began their transition from an active lifestyle with a diverse and natural diet to a lifestyle that was sedentary and a diet of limited variety and higher-calorie foods. As a result, humanity, apart from the !Kung and other hunter/gatherer outcrops, has been on a downward spiral of increasingly unhealthy living.

Ancient Greeks said that the ability to cultivate crops was given to them as a gift by the benevolent goddess Demeter. The consequence of this gift was all of the civilization, science, cities, and monuments we've produced as a species to date. But Demeter's blessing was a mixed one—agriculture enabled humans to focus on more elevated activities like science and philosophy by reducing the amount of time we had to dedicate to food procurement, but it also removed us from the way we were designed to eat. Slowly, from the Neolithic Age onward, we humans have done away with the traditional mode of foraging for plant foods and hunting for animal foods. This disconnect from our natural processes is harmful to our health in many ways and recently, humans have been paying the price for eating in a manner contrary to how we were designed. The skyrocketing obesity rates, incessant food allergies, ubiquitous prescription drugs, and persistent unhappiness throughout the population can all be attributed to the simple fact that we are not eating how we were designed.

The Evolution Diet can help. It is a painstakingly developed, yet astonishingly easy-to-follow method of getting back to your natural, healthy self. All you really need to do to become a healthier, happier person is to follow The Four Principles of The Evolution Diet: 1. Listen to your body, not your culture, 2. Appropriate your diet in the method of our ancestors, 3. Eat from nature and avoid intake of Artificially Extreme Foods (AEFs) like fried Twinkies, and 4. Exercise and sleep when your body tells you to. These steps are as simple as they are healthy but not too many people in today's society are able to overcome the cultural minutia that keeps us in a trap of unhealthy eating habits. This book will explain how you can achieve your dietetic and physical goals in easy, common sense steps. In no time at all, you will be losing weight, feeling more energetic, and sleeping better.

Many readers may find the above goals seemingly impossible to attain. If that describes you — if the idea of a truly healthy lifestyle seems so unachievable that you've almost given up or turned to prescription drugs or body-altering surgery, you've been listening to the wrong people. It's time to escape from the negative, unhealthy lifestyle you may be used to and it's time to evolve into the person you were designed to be.

Was It Something I Ate?

I'd like to begin with a story from a couple of our first trial dieters. It's possible that you will be able to identify with them as you learn of their struggles in dieting. You can be assured that since learning healthy techniques described in this book, these folks have become avid Evolution Dieters and are now living refreshingly healthy lives.

Bob was one of the first to try the Evolution Diet to help him attain a completely healthy lifestyle. He had always pictured himself as a healthy person all his life, but he had never been able to keep a consistent, healthy diet. He had played sports and had been physically active for his entire adult life, rarely going a couple of days without exercise. However, he figured that since he was exercising, he could eat anything he wanted and in whatever manner that pleased him. He went from eating large, fat-saturated Taco Bell lunches, four times per week in high school, to eating absolutely nothing all day between breakfast and dinner during his professional life. He would eat four-course meals for brunch in college and, on top of that, wolf down a full pizza at 3 A.M. after a night out!

Bob was active, probably more so than his average cohorts, but he was not healthy. His diet was unbalanced and not nutritious, and the consequences were blatant. He was slightly overweight and had such inconsistent spurts of energy and fatigue that it was debilitating. Bob was rearing to go in the morning hours when he got to work, but by mid-morning, he was practically falling asleep at his desk. Eventually, his evening sleep patterns were affected and he found himself, like 70 percent of Americans, suffering from poor sleep. He was tired during work and restless at night. Exercising helped reduce the effects of his thoughtless diet by helping reduce blood pressure and burning more calories than he would have otherwise, but eating poorly did take a toll—his ability to exercise was reduced by malnutrition, as was his interest in doing it in the first place.

Hindsight is always 20/20, so it seems obvious that Bob could have been leading a much more productive and happy life if he had just paid a little more attention to what he was eating. Eventually Bob dabbled in eating methods (he didn't want to call them diets) that were *supposed* to make him healthier.

At an early consultation we discussed his eating habits and his typical meals. He assumed there was nothing wrong with his breakfast—a regular helping of cereal—but when we analyzed it, he was shocked to discover how much sugar and how little nutrition was in his favorite cereal brands and in the 16 oz glass of orange juice he tossed back in addition. Mistakenly, he figured there couldn't be anything wrong with orange juice since it was all-natural, and the little crunchy cereal bits he was eating were fine because at least they *resembled* fruit. Although he didn't make the connection, his high-sugar breakfast was setting him up for a long day of inconsistent energy levels and hunger. When he would get to work shortly after his breakfast and just sit at his desk, he was wired and irritable and couldn't focus. Were these stressors a result of an inability to handle sitting at a desk in an office all day, or were they due to the fact that Bob wasn't eating what he was designed to eat?

Our friend Bob is an experimental type and, in the months before we met, he decided to make changes to his diet to see if that would help him feel better. First, he focused on getting rid of the nasty vending machine food that he ate for lunch, and he replaced it with a 1300-calorie veggie burrito from Rojello's Mexican restaurant down the street. This Bowling-ball-in-your-stomach-food-coma-after-lunch Diet, however appealing it may have seemed to Bob, did not work to balance his energy either.

Since that didn't work, he tried a second method to get healthier, which consisted of eliminating all food after breakfast until he got home from work. This might seem crazy to some, but Bob was confounded at the fact that he exercised nearly every day, but was still slightly overweight. Doctors wouldn't have considered him obese, but he had about 10-15 extra pounds and it was uncomfortable for him. Bob was willing to try anything and at that time, the midday fast seemed like an okay idea.

Bob was proud of his fasting diet at first. He said he probably lost some weight initially, but his energy was more inconsistent than ever and he felt like passing out by the end of the workday. Believe it or not, with such a decrease in caloric intake, Bob ended up gaining weight! Needless to say, this eating method didn't last very long.

Another early Evolution Dieter, Susan, had tried the high-protein diet and its spin-offs, with some success in losing weight, but eventually they resulted in a horrible failure in her attempts to feel better and to have more energy. Susan figured the high protein diet, was just boring her into weight loss. "I could only eat certain things and after a while I didn't feel like eating those same things, so I ate less. Not to mention, I barely had enough energy to make it through a large steak after a couple months on the diet."

After that, she took a different approach: she had a small protein breakfast and a couple snacks around midday. These snacks tended to be extremely dense and highly sugary foods (mainly dried fruit trail mix and energy bars). Although Susan wasn't *gaining* any weight, she said it seemed like she was at an all-time irritability high. In addition, when she didn't have food for any extended period, she would begin to shut down in a mild version of the condition termed hypoglycemia (low blood sugar).

Neither of these candidates, Bob or Susan, was healthy before the Evolution Diet, but they could not figure out why they

Case Study: Morena
Age:46 Goal: Weight loss

The most astonishing thing about the Evolution Diet to Morena was the fact that just by altering the time when she ate certain foods, she lost weight.

"I ate about the same amount of food I normally was eating, maybe even more, but I lost weight from eating all my carbs throughout the day and all my proteins at night. It was amazing to see the pounds drop from just that!"

Morena learned the most basic aspect to The Evolution Diet: not only is it important to eat healthy foods, it's important to eat certain foods at certain times.

There's a place for almost every type of food you can imagine in The Evolution Diet, but one must eat them at the appropriate time. For instance, Morena always had a craving for buttered popcorn. She would usually cook up a batch in the late evening, about an hour before sleep. What she didn't realize was that she was filling herself with mostly carbohydrates and fat and not using those calories immediately because she was going to sleep.

All of these extra calories went straight to her waistline as stored fat. When she moved her popcorn 'meal' to the daytime, the weight came off almost immediately.

were *un*healthy considering they were both eating so-called "health foods". They got to the point where they were eating pretty much all natural foods and both were eating moderate proportions with regard to hunger—they were not stuffing their faces—and they were only eating when they were hungry. They just could not figure out why they felt so unhealthy. This is when they decided to contact a nutritional specialist and learn how to become truly healthy.

I took them on as studies and set them on a plan of eating and exercising that has become the Evolution Diet.

Background of the Diet

If you've eaten a California sushi roll, delighted in strawberry yogurt, or had a Shirley Temple cocktail recently, you probably ingested a peculiar ingredient that you weren't aware of. The ingredient comes from the cochineal beetle, a parasitic insect that lives on cacti and produces a rich red dye called carmine, which is used in imitation crabmeat, strawberry yogurt, and maraschino cherries. The dye derived from the beetle is usually listed as an "artificial color," which sounds harmless enough, but it can generate a rare, yet potentially fatal, allergic reaction.

This illustration shows something remarkable about our eating culture: most of us don't have any clue what we're really putting into our bodies. I certainly didn't pay attention to the ingredients I was engulfing in processed foods during my formative years. I figured, it's on the shelf at the store or billions of people are eating it (as in the case of McDonald's), it must be okay. Of course, this is an extremely misguided perspective, though completely understandable. We have constant influences telling us to eat this or stuff our faces with that and eating off the land has become a completely foreign concept to most of the population. The concept of a diet is nothing close to its original meaning was.

So, over a decade ago, I set out to strip away all of the cultural noise about dieting and what to eat and really find out what *and* how we really were designed to eat. What I learned was shocking, however obvious as it may seem after the fact: the average modern American diet is dramatically contrary to what we, as humans, were designed to eat. I learned that gastronomic institutions such as "three square meals" and the "balanced meal" are actually bad for us because they contradict with our natural metabolic processes. I learned that most of the foods in the typical diet have been so densely packed with processed ingredients that almost every time we eat, we are overloading our systems, which causes unnecessary, detrimental stress on our physiological systems. I also learned that some of the major staple foods that our diet relies on are detrimental to our health.

Cultural institutions like the balanced meal and marketing gimmicks like the low-carb diet have added to a painfully flawed artificial diet, which in turn, has lead to a physically ill society. But, in response to the nation's ailments like obesity, high blood pressure, and heart problems, the medical establishment's answer has typically been a moneymaking prescription drug of some sort, not sound nutritional advice. Should you expect any different? Doctors make their livings off of people when they're sick and ordering their heavily pushed pharmaceuticals, not when they're healthy. This is a tragic situation and one that should be accompanied with a sizeable amount of skepticism toward the dietetic industry in general. I, on the other hand, do not own a white coat or a stethoscope and I am not lobbied by Big Pharma. It is not my goal to convince you that a magic pill that may do more harm than good is the answer and charge you for it. What I intend to offer with The Evolution Diet is a common sense dietetic assessment of where we came from, where we are now, and where we should be going. And the cost of this book is much less than the price of that little white pill or stomach stapling surgery!

Through tireless research and study, I've developed a plan for eating which takes into account two factors of modern food variety (personal and cultural influences) and our very own natural processes. The Evolution Diet is not just a way to effectively lose weight, but also a plan for maintaining a perfectly healthy lifestyle

 An Evolution Diet Essential

There is a middle ground in weight which the human body is perfectly content. It is a natural state of being, in which the calories ingested are equivalent to the calories expended and which there is no excess fat. This is the goal.

for your entire life while avoiding detrimental food allergens. In addition, when you eat the way you were designed to eat, you will not only achieve your ideal weight, but you will feel energetic when you should, sleepy when it's time, and generally healthier throughout the day. Sounds good doesn't it?

The major problem with today's lifestyle is that we've gotten too far away from our natural diet while letting culture force its will on our physiology. The results are scary: widespread depression, sleeplessness, fatigue, and, of course, obesity. Even for people who are not overweight, diet is integral to overall health. If you have been feeling inexplicable irritability, sadness, fatigue, loss in alertness, or just lack of good health, the latest pharmaceutical pill is NOT the answer! It's quite possible that a return to natural eating patterns is the only thing you'll need. If you alter what you eat, and equally importantly, *how* you eat, just a bit, you may be on the way to living a perfectly healthy, and happy life. Take control of your life—it's time to evolve!

A Brief Overview of the Diet

The Evolution Diet is revolutionary not because it uses cutting-edge chemistry, but rather because it uses ancient biology. It encourages you to get more in touch with your body and know how it was designed to eat. It also encourages you to eat how and when you were meant to eat, not just what you were meant to eat. When this happens, you will eat the types of food you would without the influences of culture and regain the ideal weight you may have previously lost. This will inevitably lead to a happier, healthier life all around.

One of the unique aspects of The Evolution Diet: All-Natural and Allergy Free is that it is a consistent plan for eating throughout one's life. While most other diets start participants off with a "shock-your-system" introduction followed by eating in moderation, The Evolution Diet calls for one unique, life-long method of eating, which reflects your personal lifestyle and can support you through activity or inactivity.

The goal is to imitate the diet of natural humans (or, as referred to onward as Natural Man or Nat) in order to fit the diet our bodies have been designed to take in. Regardless of how you think our species was designed, we were made to eat certain things and in a certain way. Natural Man (without present culture) had been around 500 times longer than Cultural Man and his extremely efficient and excessively caloric foods. During all that time, our ancestors' digestive systems were selected to eat based on our surroundings and environment, which varies only slightly outside of the Arctic Circle.

In essence, Natural Man evolved to eat a specific way: small quantities of low-sugar and high-fiber foods (referred to in this book as LoS Hi-Fi foods) throughout the day until he hunted and subsequently gorged on mass quantities of nutritious, lean meat. This simplified version of the subsistence hunter/gatherer diet illustrates a rough outline of the foods our bodies are expecting us to feed it. If we don't feed our bodies a diet along those lines, they react adversely with the conditions like weight gain, heart problems, and sleep apnea, and which eventually send some to the doctor's office.

The Evolution Diet begins with the basic hunter/gatherer diet and infuses a modern diversity of foods and exercise to produce the most well-rounded, sophisticated dietetic plan yet. Optimal wellbeing can be obtained by combining the intrinsic wisdom of our genes with the wealth and expertise of today.

If you enjoy eating—and who doesn't?—then you will enjoy The Evolution Diet. On the whole, people eat more with the techniques in this book than they did before, yet they achieve their ideal weight and keep to it. To answer that sudden 'How do they do that?' question that popped in your head, look at The Evolution Diet as a way to work *with* your body, and not against it like so many modern diets do. When we eat the way we were designed, we use our bodies' natural mechanics to work for us by keeping our metabolism at a constant high and the higher our metabolism is, the more energy we need to keep it running.

But it's important to understand that eating shouldn't be the ultimate goal in life. A simple concept that is lost in today's consumer-driven society is that eating is good for humans because it helps us live, not because it feels good. Unfortunately, we live in a culture that twists our natural urges and practically forces us to eat things contrary to our nature. Sugar and fat helped our ancestors survive to reproduce and thus, we evolved to like the taste of those things. Sugar and fat, however, were rare in the Stone Age and only recently have they become overly abundant in our diet. Today, food scientists have exploited our natural liking for sugar and fat and present our watering mouths with fried Twinkies and 64-ounce Big Gulps, which we did not evolve to ingest. The goal is to return to the tasty, healthy foods you were actually designed to eat and, in doing so, be able to eat more of them while still achieving an ideal weight.

Besides eating, we humans can amuse ourselves quite thoroughly. We can play games, sing, write poetry, build Channel Tunnels and Hoover Dams, explore our universe and most importantly, we can educate our young. Notwithstanding the distinct art that culinary science is, eating should be seen as a means to do all of those other things, instead of the goal of life itself. Eating should make our bodies happy, and, in turn, make our minds happy. As Cicero once said, "One should eat to live, not live to eat."

The Evolution Diet doesn't tell you to shun foods that taste good, but rather how to fit them into a healthy diet. You'll find too that upon adjusting your diet to a healthier, more natural one, even the ordinary foods available to us that used to taste so bland and uninteresting have plenty of flavors waiting to please your taste buds—it is possible to actually crave broccoli! This book will describe that method and help you get to that place.

I will describe how our bodies were designed over the course of evolution, which will give us clues as to what we should be eating. Then I will take a lighter, and often unappetizing look at how culture influences our diet and contrast that with a culture-less, natural diet. It is vital for us to understand what goes on in our bodies, at least to some extent, so I will then describe our bodies' chemistry and how it reacts to the main macronutrients: carbohydrates, proteins, and fats and show how some popular foods today work against our evolved physiology.

With all of the background information presented, I will describe, in depth, the Evolution Diet: All-Natural and Allergy Free, what and how exactly you should be eating to match your modern lifestyle, and more importantly, to match how you were designed to eat. I will also describe tips on how to emulate Natural Man and broaden your dietary menu with a variety of wild plants. The positive results of returning to a more natural Evolution Diet will be self-evident, but in the last Part I will foreshadow those by giving you the physical reactions to look for while Evo-dieting. First, though, I would like to contest the current notion of diet and explain what a diet really should be seen as.

The Purpose of a Diet

Ever since certain fad diets became popular in the seventies and eighties, the general conception of a 'diet' is viewed as a quick and easy tool to help its participants lose a few pounds, without any regard to lifelong eating habits. In other words, it is seen as a short-term fix. What ends up happening with people on these short-term plans is that they tend to go back to eating poorly after the weight goal has been met or worse, when the weight goal hasn't been met and seems impossible to achieve. In fact, researchers at UCLA have recently revealed shocking findings: dieting just doesn't work. The school reviewed 31 long-term studies on dieting and found that people who go on diets usually end up regaining all of the weight they lost, plus some after they stop dieting. In addition to the weight gain, researchers say that the ups and downs of dieting cause added stress and contribute to heart disease. The study seems bleak for those looking to shed pounds, but, still, people continue the quick-fix methods, moving to the next one as soon as they give up on the previous one, usually to no avail.

This yo-yo dieting confuses the body and frustrates the psyche, and never quite lives up to the sensational claims that these diet gimmicks advertise. Testimonials similar to, "I lost 50 pounds in 5 weeks!" and "I dropped 15 pounds the first week!" lead to inaccurate interpretations of what a diet should be. If these people were to continue on their so-called diet, they would be weightless within a couple years. Now that would be amazing!

The truth is that these diets, which temporarily allow rapid weight loss, are often times just dehydrating the body. The weight lost on these diets is primarily in H_2O not LBS, and since the body is about 60 percent water, it is fairly easy to drop a few pounds of it. Inevitably, though, the 'contestants' on these 'miracle diets' must change their habits back or at least alter them so as not to eliminate themselves from existence altogether.

These whacky eating habits are missing the point completely and they are leading to a misnomer. A diet, by definition, is not some two-week panacea to help you lose weight; it is much broader than just that. A diet is someone's general intake of food. People still have a diet even when they're not *on* a diet. A diet also is something that takes place over one's entire life, not just the five weeks before one's wedding day or class reunion. When looked at in this light, people who go on those gimmicky diets advertised on late-night television aren't on a high-protein diet, or a lettuce-only plan; these people are on an extremely unhealthy yo-yo diet.

Changing one's eating habits so drastically so often is bad for one's health, something that most diet promoters fail to explain. Interestingly, an obese person has a better chance of living longer than someone who fluctuates habitually between being obese and having an ideal weight. A University of Michigan study conducted by cardiologist Claire Duvernoy, M.D. has found that a direct link between the gain-loss-gain syndrome of yo-yo dieting and cardiovascular disease in women. It turns out that such an oscillation of weight adds a great deal more stress than a constant weight. But Natural Man went through long droughts without food — doesn't that mean that we are designed to withstand ups and downs in our diet like our ancestors? While we do have a remarkable capability to adapt to our environment (described further in Part Two), up-and-down dieting is still considerably harmful. In addition, during a drought, Natural Man's body mass index (BMI) shifted from ideal to underweight and back — a completely different physiological story than a BMI that shifts from obese to overweight and back.

That isn't to say that one shouldn't try to lose weight if they're a little tight in the waistline. The constantly obese person has a drastically smaller chance of living longer than someone at a constant ideal weight. A Dutch study published in the *Annals of Internal Medicine* (2003) says that obese women live an average of 7.1 fewer years than women of normal weight. Obese men live 5.8 fewer years on average than their healthy counterparts. That's almost 10 percent of the average lifespan!

The solution for everyone is to learn a method of eating that brings everyone to his or her ideal weight and keeps them there without the need to yo-yo diet. The typical counter to that statement would be, "Well, everyone is different. There can't possibly be a diet that works for everyone." But there is. It just so happens that at one point, all humans did eat the same diet: the natural hunter/gatherer diet, and they were remarkably healthier than we are today despite lack of medicine and wealth as we'll see later. The Evolution Diet emulates this healthy hunter/gatherer diet and supports a robust lifestyle for everyone, regardless of personality or physical makeup. Because this method of eating is strictly linked to the natural methods of the body, it will work to create a stable, healthy weight for everyone who adheres to the guidelines. One of the most vital attributes of The Evolution Diet is that it is even beneficial for people who are already at their ideal weights, thus someone can maintain just one diet for their entire life, the healthy way it should be.

What about the fat gene? Some people would argue that some people were born with a 'fat gene,' and it is nearly impossible for those people to maintain a healthy weight without surgery or medical assistance in the form of prescription drugs. It is understandable if you have accepted this train of thought since it pervades the popular media. There are people out there that want to make you think that you have no say in your physical state. . . ah, but their *magical* pill does. The FDA does not recognize any form of natural cure (i.e. exercise or antioxidants) as a treatment for disease. Only artificial drugs can be called a treatment and this seems a little suspect to me.

It just so happens that there is very little that differs between humans, with respect to genes, even when it comes to a person's weight or retention of fat. A recent study conducted by Dr. Roy J. Britten at the California Institute of Technology (published in *Proceedings of the National Academy of Sciences*) has found that even humans and chimpanzees have nearly identical genetic makeup. According to the study, 95 percent of the genetic makeup of chimps is the same as that of humans. Shockingly, we're even quite similar to plants like a pumpkin. Similar methods of experimentation showed that pumpkins and humans share about 75 percent of our DNA. However, this doesn't mean we need to look like a pumpkin!

Based on the study's findings, it appears that just being

alive accounts for so much of our genetic code, that there is very little left over to produce differences like eating tendencies or nuances in the digestive system. The CIT study has found that two different humans are 99.9 percent genetically identical. Based on the number of genes scientists have found that humans have (about 30,000), you are only 30 or so genes different from Mick Jagger and this applies to everyone with the normal amount of 23 paired chromosomes. That's astounding.

It turns out that our previous idea of a gene for every protein created was the wrong way to think about it. It's not the number of genes that determines who we are, but what our genes do with what they are given that gives us the diversity and complexity of being human. So we can actually alter what our genes do and how they work based on what we feed them. In other words, we truly are what we eat. Likewise, the perception that genetic makeup determines who we are is also false. It is what we *do* with our genetic makeup that makes us who we are.

This stirs up the ancient argument of Nature versus Nurture, which to my knowledge has not been definitively answered. No one can deny we are products of our genes—just think of all the times you've heard, "You've got your father's eyes," or more unfortunately, "You've got your father's bald patch." But even the most ardent Naturalists will concede that behavior plays a significant role in one's physical construction. They would add that all people could be fit and healthy, though they would argue that some people need to try harder than others for ideal health. I contest that it's not a matter of trying harder, but rather being more thoughtful and simply living how we were designed to live. Thus, without going into the argument of Nature versus Nurture, we must presume that regardless of one's genetic makeup, everyone can be lean and fit. No one is precluded from attaining a healthy body and a healthy mind (with an ideal weight).

This is one of the most important factors in achieving a healthy lifestyle: You must know that you can do it for it to be possible at all. The beneficial aspects of positive psychology are unlimited, and though the idea is important to understand, it deserves its own book and I can't do it justice here. Instead, here's a list of clichés that illustrate the benefits of positive thinking:

- "You can't achieve anything without trying."
- "A negative attitude will get you nowhere."
- "The luckiest people tend to be the ones who always work harder."
- "Nothing valuable comes without a price."
- "Haste makes waste."
- "When life gives you lemons, make lemonade."
- "Turn that frown upside down." (This one doesn't really apply, but it's nice anyway.)

With that little bit of motivation, perhaps the reader can better understand the idea that we're all made with basically the same instructions, but we don't all do the same thing with those instructions. I've heard countless times people say that it is *impossible* to be as thin as a supermodel or some famous skinny actress. On the contrary, it is extremely likely for anyone to be that thin if they did the same things. This is based on one simple principle: if someone expends more calories than he takes in, he will lose weight, and if he takes in more calories than he burns, he will gain weight. This applies to average Joe as much as it applies to Cindy Crawford or Gisele Bündchen. What my acquaintances and others mean to say when they scoff at the impossible supermodels is that, "It's impossible to be as thin as those models while eating what I eat and exercising as little as I do." When it's phrased that way, it seems kind of obvious, doesn't it?

It is important to note that the idea here is not to be bone-thin; in fact, super-thin supermodels are probably not as healthy as they could be because some fat is necessary for a completely healthy body to operate (we will discuss this in Part Four). The important thing is to be healthy, which certainly includes not being overweight, but also includes not being underweight. There are equally detrimental problems associated with being underweight as there are with being overweight, although, in today's American society, the former is not as prevalent of a problem. It is also common to maintain a constant body weight while exercising and eating proportionally, yet, to still have an unhealthy body weight.

There is a middle ground in weight at which the human body is perfectly content. It is a natural state of being, in which the calories ingested are equivalent to the calories expended and which there is no excess storage of calories to maintain. This is the state that we should want to achieve—a state that is free from culturally influenced abnormalities such as three square meals per day, the gigantic-sized portions of take-out culture, Atkins, the cabbage diet, and fast food. The healthy, natural state is a condition of existence, which your body has been begging you to achieve for all of your life. Your body has told you when you are not treating it right with uncomfortable feelings like guilt, perhaps some health conditions, and even pain.

It is time that you rid yourself of all that negativity issued by an unhealthy diet and to move to a clean and healthy method of eating. It's time to get to the state of perfect balance within yourself, to start listening to your body and become the healthy individual you know you can be. It is time to evolve.

Part Two
How We Evolved
(The Omnivore Debate)

Q: What do you call a fake noodle?
A: An iMPASTA!

"You know you are dieting when stamps start to taste good."

-Anonymous

In the late afternoon of an East African savannah 3.6 million years ago, two animals went for a stroll. A nearby volcano had just erupted placing a layer of ash on the ground and a slight rain had made a cement-like paste of the ash. When the animals passed through a particular area of the savannah, now called Laetoli, their footprints were captured in the paste and hardened before another plum of ash blanketed the area again. Those footprints were not seen again until 1976, when Mary Leakey's team of paleontologists uncovered them while working in Tanzania. The remarkable thing about those footprints is that when Mary Leakey first spotted them, she identified them as human prints—the animals that left the tracks were strolling upright on two legs that afternoon.

Besides significant physical record of the fossils, the footprints also leave unmistakable evidence of human-like behavior. The two animals were walking close together—likely holding each other—and at one point the smaller of the two (probably a female) hesitated in her stride, turned left to glance at a possible threat, then continued in the original direction. These observations of humanistic behaviors in addition to discoveries of nearby fossils have lead scientists to determine that the prehistoric walkers were ancestors of modern Homo sapiens—a species called Australopithecus afarensis.

It was this species that made the giant leap from tree-dwelling fruit and insect eaters to hunter/gatherers that dominated the food chain. Some time before the aforementioned fossilized stroll occurred, the climate in Africa began to change. Dry and rainy seasons were introduced and the jungle in which Australopithecus' ancestors lived slowly evaporated, leaving wide-open savannahs spotted with clumps of acacia trees. Species that were able to adapt to the new climate survived—others didn't. As for A. afarensis, walking on two legs (or bipedalism) freed their hands to allow them to carry food to their camps and away from danger. Walking upright also reduced the amount of skin that was exposed to the sun, which ultimately helped save afarensis from heat stroke and allowed them to travel long distances at a time. Without bipedalism, A. afarensis wouldn't have been as successful of a species as it was and might not have survived in such a dynamic environment.

As the chain of evolution progressed from A. afarensis to A. africanus to Homo habilis to Homo erectus and on to Homo sapiens, the hunter/gatherer lifestyle was perfected and improved upon. Early Homo sapiens were the beneficiaries of millions of years of evolution, which allowed them to adapt to a wide variety

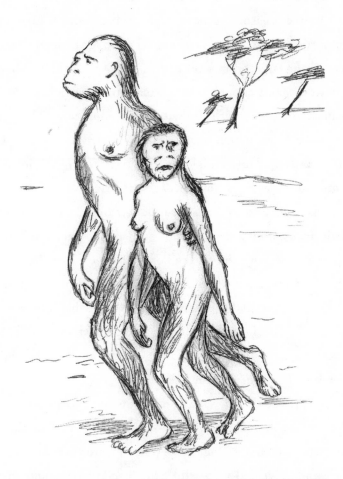

The hunter/gatherer lifestyle began with the bipedal Australopithecus afarensis in what is now East Africa.

of climates and environments. In fact, our species has been able to expand prolifically from a group of about 40,000 in Central Africa, to nearly 7 billion covering the entire globe. We have acclimated to most of the climates on Earth: barren deserts in the Americas to the bitter cold tundra of Northern Asia. We have been able to survive where other animals could not (forest, savannah, and mountains) and we're able to sit at the top of the food chain despite our species' lack of natural defense mechanisms, like claws or horns.

Another reason we have been so successful in dominating our surroundings and rocketing to the top of the food chain is because of our large brain size. Even before modern technology, humans were smart enough to catch or trap larger animals, or to find fruits and vegetables that other animals could not. The !Kung San from the Introduction have an ability in tracking their prey that many anthropologists think trace back to the dawn of man. In being able to understand how recent hoof prints were made and where those prints led to the animal that created them, the !Kung and their ancestors had an enormous advantage over the lion or other predator seeking dinner. If a lion didn't see the wildebeest in the distance, it could not start licking its chops, but the large brains of the first humans enabled them to garner valuable information from a few imprints in the ground. So, a large portion of credit for our success as a species should go to whoever thought of giving us a large brain. That was brilliant!

But besides being smart and knowing how to find prey when other hungry animals couldn't, we humans have a number of *digestive* traits and abilities that make it possible for us to be so evolutionarily adaptive and successful. Our species has useful natural tools such as sharp canine teeth and highly acidic digestive juices, which may not seem like much, but which allow us to digest the proteins that our bodies need from certain foods. Vegetarians will instantly refute this as an archaic remnant of a barbarous path of mammalian existence: the carnivore. But those teeth needed to cut meat and the acids in our stomachs exist because it was evolutionarily beneficial for our ancestors to eat nutritious meat. What we should do with those traits now are still up for debate.

In addition to our beneficial teeth and stomach fluids, we

have a digestive system that, shocking as it may sound, contains billions of helper animals which help break down foods to give us the nutrients that we need. Like it or not, we require bacteria to digest our food, without which, we would not be able to survive. We are lucky that our bodies have chosen to be nice and allow those bacteria to remain in the Small Intestine Hotel instead of trying to kill them off like malicious intruders.

Another handy feature we have is our single stomach, which helps us maintain a relatively small abdomen and allows us to walk upright, instead of requiring four legs to hold us up. A cow has 4 different chambers in its stomach system, all of which are needed to digest the food it eats (mainly grass). Can you image having to walk around with 75 gallons of additional stomach space in your body? Not to mention having to regurgitate food that we've already eaten just to chew it back up and send it back through. We are lucky to have our one stomach, which can break up almost anything it comes in contact with.

All of these features that the human body has leads to one result: the ability to eat a wide variety of foods efficiently. Before explaining why this is a benefit to us as animals, I will describe the omnivore debate and explain the clues that lead me to believe we are naturally omnivorous.

In the class mammalia, there are vegetarians and meat-eaters. Which one of those Homo sapiens are naturally has been a matter of debate since the beginning of history. Most anthropologists and doctors place us in the category of omnivore; however, many plant-eaters and strict meat-eaters among us have tried very hard to convince people that that name is inaccurate.

In determining whether an animal is herbivorous (strictly plant eating), frugivorous (mainly fruit eating), carnivorous (strictly meat eating), or omnivorous (eats just about anything), it is important to critique the tools used to come to a determination. It is not good enough to say that humans are omnivorous because you see people eat a salad before dinner and a steak during dinner. Observation doesn't make for a complete study. I've seen a human being eat metal nails and screws, but that doesn't quite make it natural, healthy, or especially logical.

Many types of eating habits result in or from distinct physical characteristics. And using the physical characteristics that humans have and comparing those with the characteristics of animals in each eating type, we should be able to divulge the answer to the question: what should we be eating?

Oral Cavity

For most carnivores (picture man's best friend, the dog), the oral cavity, or mouth, is wide with spaced-out teeth, so as to prevent the stringy things in meat from sticking around and to avoid the times when we would use floss to get at them. The incisors in carnivores are short and prong-like. They are used to grip onto prey. The canines are long and dagger like, used to stab and tear flesh. When the jaw of a carnivore closes, the teeth in the back come together like a pair of scissors in order to produce an effective cutting action.

Herbivores, on the other hand, don't need such cutting and slicing or tearing and stabbing. An herbivore's prey is pretty defenseless, because their prey is plant life. All an herbivore needs to get its food into its stomach is a grinding mechanism. Herbivores' teeth are flatter and do not slide past one another to create a scissor-like cutting action. Some herbivores, like pigs, have enormous canines, but unlike their carnivorous distant cousins, these teeth are usually not used for hunting prey, but rather as a defense mechanism as in the case of the ancient wild boar. Some herbivores don't even have canines at all, or instead, just a bottom pair, as in the case of our friendly cow.

One important difference between most carnivores and most herbivores is the composition of their saliva. In most herbivores, there is an enzyme (amylase) that aids in the digestion of carbohydrates, so that food digestion starts happening once the animal takes a bite. Carnivores, on the other hand, do not produce this enzyme. They wait for the food to get to their stomach to start digestion and when the carnivore is good at what it does, it doesn't take very long to get the flesh into the stomach. After the meat-eater kills its prey, it gorges itself and retreats away from the battleground to digest, wary of reprisals from other animals. Herbivores, like elephants aren't going to be hurried by anyone, since their food is so abundant and not difficult to capture. They can take their time and grind up their food right where they found it.

Digestive Tract

The differences between carnivores and herbivores with regard to their digestive tract are far more reaching and elaborate. To begin, carnivores have one stomach and very low pH level inside of it (around pH 1). This means that the environment in a carnivore's stomach is very acidic. The intensely acidic mixture of chemicals is needed to break apart the proteins in the meat. Additionally, the acid is used to kill off the detrimental bacteria, which thrive on flesh open to the air. The stomach in most carnivores is widely expandable in order to allow for large quantities of food in short amounts of time. Also, the small intestine is substantially shorter in carnivores.

Good thing we don't have a cow's digestive tract!

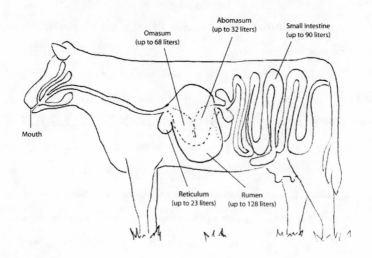

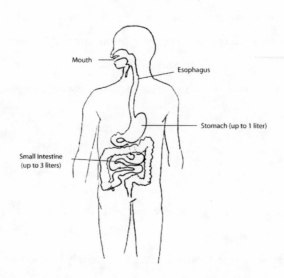

Herbivores, as mentioned before, may have multiple stomachs, which are needed for the longer digestion of the plants they eat. Strict herbivores (bovines for instance) have stomach capacities 150 times that of an average human's and their food sits in the digestive tract for considerably longer amounts of time. To fully break down the cells in grass, for instance, to obtain the intracellular goodies, herbivores must let the mass of plants they've eaten ferment in their digestive tract. This process of fermentation occurs when bacteria breaks down the substance for the host animal. Those herbivores that do not ferment cellulose (the fiber found in much of plant life) usually get their nutrition from more easily digested soft vegetation, like fruits and vegetables.

A Mixed Bag

As you can see with the comparisons between herbivores' and carnivores' physical makeup, they are extremely different, and it shouldn't be hard to determine which group of animals we humans belong in. We should be able to place our characteristics into one of the two categories (meat-eater, or plant-eater). However, it turns out that humans are a mixed bag of physical digestive traits.

Humans have many flat teeth that do not slide past one another (molars), and which are perfect for grinding up plants, but also have a full set of sharp canines, which, depending on your amount of overbite or underbite, do slide past one another in a slicing fashion. This diastema, or space between the canine teeth, allow for the sharper teeth to make the scissor-like motion. They aren't very long canines, which means that we do not use them as weapons for attacking or defense and the fact that we do not need our teeth for weapons means that the chewing capability is the only determinant factor.

We produce the same enzyme in our saliva that herbivores do in order to begin digestion immediately, but the stomach of a human can be extremely acidic, pH 1, which lends itself nicely to digesting meat (as will be described further in Part Four).

It has also been noted that a high intake of dense plant

carbohydrates, which has happened since the inception of farming, has also decreased oral health, including more dental carries. This could mean that eating highly caloric plant carbohydrates the way we do today is not natural and doesn't fit with how we were designed.

The time it takes to digest food for humans is relatively small compared with strict herbivores. This is because we can get our protein from sources other than plants, so we don't need to let the food sit in our stomachs for hours on end, only to regurgitate it and swallow it again to let it simmer in the stomach pools some more just to extract the protein from grass. Rather, we can get our protein from meat (where the protein is much more readily available), and all we need to take from the plants are their vitamins and energy (which are fairly easy to extract from plants).

Although we have many characteristics of a plant-eater, the fact that we digest things so quickly makes it necessary for humans to eat meat in order to take in everything we need, most notably protein. According to a recent paper by an anthropologist DJ Chivers, "Humans are on the inner edge of the faunivore cluster, showing the distinctive adaptations of their guts for meat-eating, or for some other rapidly digested foods, in contrast to the frugivorous apes (and monkeys)."

Something else that separates us from our plant-eating cousins is our relatively small digestive tract compared to strict herbivores, which require warehouses of storage in order to digest what they eat. Most primates are mainly fruit-eaters, but have omnivorous leanings; for instance, chimpanzees have a keen liking for ants, which tend to have a lot of protein, but do not require sharp teeth to eat. Chimps also have a taste for small animals like mice, bush pigs, and squirrels. Other primates, such as the ground-dwelling baboons, who live in the open country, seem to be particularly good at hunting small game as well as insects. These cousins of ours have been known to easily surround infant gazelles and antelopes, kill, and consume them.

One advantage humans have over many animals is our extremely adjustable mandible (jaw). The fact that it can move back and forth and side to side makes for the potential of a complete diet. No matter what the food is and regardless of our dental makeup, we can chew our food in such a way as to simulate a carnivore or an herbivore.

Another possible dietetic advantage that we have as humans is our eyesight. It just so happens that the most vividly colored foods are the ones with the most to offer with respect to vitamins and nutrient density. Have you ever heard the rule of thumb that the greener the lettuce, the better it is for you? Compare the bark of a tree and the nearby orange hanging from it. To the human eye, the orange will stand out dramatically and thus will attract us more. It is not just a coincidence that the orange is better for you too. The National Cancer Institute (NCI), which has recently launched a campaign to promote foods by their bright colors called, "Savor the Spectrum" suggests that foods with brighter colors contain more nutrients and one must cover the entire spectrum to get all the nutrients one needs. Now, we not only have a food pyramid to pay attention to, we also have a color wheel to think of. According to NCI, eating lush greens provides the phytonutrients (nutrients from a plant) leutin and indoles; orange foods provide beta-carotene and bioflavinoids; reds give you lycopene and anthocyanins; blues/purples provide anthocyanins phenolics; and white foods give us allicin. Each phytonutrient provides unique benefits including reducing the risk of cancer, boosting immunity, and helping skin, eyesight, and heart health among other benefits.

Since we can see the color that attracts us to such healthy

nutrients, a diet of brilliantly colored red tomatoes, orange carrots, yellow lemons, green broccoli, and blue blueberries put us way ahead of man's best color-blind friend, the dog. The dog, since it is a meat-eater, focuses on motion as opposed to color in deciding what to eat. You've maybe heard that dogs are color blind—their eyes have evolved that way to hunt active prey, not pick out vibrant fruits and vegetables from surrounding foliage. But we humans can spot an orange or a bunch or blueberries and we're healthier for it.

How a Dynamic Physiology Helps Humans

It's all well and good that we are physically capable of eating just about any type of nourishment, but does that actually benefit us, and if so, how does it benefit us? A dynamic physiology with regard to diet does help us out as a species for one reason in particular: if one source of food is suddenly taken away from our menu, we have alternatives to fall back on. If we relied on just one food source and that was taken away from us, we would surely suffer from deprivation. In times of drought, for instance, common herbivores slowly die out easily because the plants that sustain them are not as readily available. But months after the plants have all died, there are still some carnivores sticking around, stubbornly, because they can get nutrition from food sources not as dependent on water. Being able to eat animals when there are no plants around is a big plus! Being omnivorous means that we humans aren't dictated by natural disasters to the extent that strict herbivores are. And when all the land animals, which have supported the humans in a drought, have been killed, there are the ocean-based animals such as fish, which can still support the group. Before modern times, of course, the wealth of animal life in the oceans was never threatened and continued to supply coastal communities with endless amounts of food.

Most of our modern physiology is the way it is because it helps us survive in a changing environment. Why did our ancestors—the Australopithecus from the beginning of this chapter—decide to walk? It wasn't because it looked fun; it was because they had to become bipedal in order to survive. Peter Wheeler of John Moores University in Liverpool has asserted that the increased exposure to the sun for those species in the open savannahs favored an upright stance, which aids in cooling the body by upwards of 60 percent. When searching or hunting for food during hot African afternoons, it was beneficial for A. afarensis to be able to walk like a human.

Not all species were as lucky as our ancestors', though. The mastodon, which roamed North America from about 1.5 million to 10,000 years ago, had a much more difficult time when the climate shifted. Mastodons dominated in the post-dinosaur era, and it was especially well suited for the cold ice age that existed at that time. When the major freeze subsided around 10,000 years ago, the elephant-like beasts, along with its cousin, the mammoth, died out. There is speculation as to why exactly the species died out, but many scientists attribute the extinction to the climate change, which affected the types of available food, thus limiting the mastodons' usual diet. The animals couldn't alter their diet and thus couldn't survive the dramatic climate change. When the mastodons and mammoths became extinct, one of their predators, the saber-toothed cat lost a major component of its diet and that species also became extinct. Humans were newcomers to the area at that time but outlived both species because of their high adaptability and their omnivorous eating habits. They didn't die out because they were able to shift their diet to match the changing environment.

Another trait that allowed our ancestors to adapt was their hunter/gatherer lifestyle, which allowed them to move from place to place to find food. Unlike settled people, hunter/gatherers could move around to avoid the consequences of drought or disease. As anthropologist Marvin Harris wrote in his summa of the human race, *Our Kind*, "Hunter-gatherers were more likely to suffer temporary food shortages, but less likely to suffer from prolonged starvation since they were highly mobile and could improve their diet by moving to areas less affected by drought and other natural disasters. Agriculturalists," he continued, "were likely to have only one hungry season per year. But from time to time their crops would fail and they would suffer prolonged famine without being able to abandon their villages and fields."

The fact that humans are omnivores allows us to survive and thrive in every part of the globe, regardless of the natural disasters that may alter the food supply. Sure, it helps to have an active and large brain to help become the most dominant species on Earth, but without the ability to eat a vastly diverse diet from different places, we may well have died out along with the mastodons and the saber-toothed cats. In this respect, we have our dynamic physiology to thank for our position on top of the food chain.

Part Three

The Cultureless Diet
(How Natural Man Would Eat)

Q: If you eat a candy bar in the forest and no one is there to see you eat it, does it have any calories?

Q: Is your idea of a balanced diet a cookie in each hand?

A new type of human has evolved on this planet recently, according to Nobel Laureate Robert Fogel. This subspecies has developed through a new type of evolution, which is not based on genes, but rather is based on the technological and physiological improvements that we have made to our environment and our bodies. Compared to 300 years ago, this new evolution has helped more people live longer and has also helped improve the quality of that longer life; but there is a major drawback to this pseudo-evolution. Since our genes haven't changed dramatically for tens of thousands of years, this modern "technophysio" evolution has presented a problem in cultures that are so technologically advanced that they are able to meet their nutritional requirements and then some. We've gone overboard in our quest to feed our insatiable appetites and the result could be seen soon in a reduction of life expectancy for people born in the next few years.

How did we come to such a state where something so vital to our existence — eating — has come to harm and endanger us? We are biologically designed to eat a certain way, yet we humans are so smart and so technologically advanced that we've gotten to the point where we can ignore what our genes want us to eat and, instead, focus on what television commercials want us to eat. Instead of choosing from a vast diet of all-natural and healthy foods from our natural geographic surroundings, we can now select from a widely varied menu of natural or unnatural; local or exotic; and healthy or unhealthy foods. For those of us in developed countries, our menu is as large as our imagination.

In addition to the abundance and variety of food, we humans have mastered the ability to invent hyper-sensitizing foods. For example, scientists have been able to make a substance that is 8,000 times as sweet as sugar. This means that to match the sweetness of 1 tablespoon of this super-sweetener (it's called neotame), you would need over 31 gallons of regular table sugar. Wow! Talk about a sensory explosion!

Although these super-sweeteners can be explained mathematically, there are also some things that modern culinary scientists have created that cannot be explained. An example is the McDonald's French fry. A regular serving of fries (a puny 4 ounces) has basically no nutritional value, but has 20 percent of the recommended daily allowance of saturated fat, trans fats, a secret *un*natural ingredient for flavor described as, "an animal source," 220 milligrams of sodium, and enough calories to save a small village from starving for a week. Besides being unhealthy, McDonald's fries are also uncanny in other ways. In Morgan Spurlock's documentary *Super-size Me*, the viewer is treated to a makeshift science experiment in which a few fast food menu items are placed in separate glass jars and observed as they rot over the course of many weeks. The burgers and fish sandwich all began to decay within days and turn into "moldy goodness" according to Spurlock, but the

 An Evolution Diet Essential

With our scientific expertise and our seemingly weak will power, we humans are straying away from what we are naturally designed to eat.

McDonald's French fries looked brand new over two months after purchase. This experiment inspires the question if bacteria and mold spores are too good for McDonald's French fries, why are we humans eating them? If the fries don't break down and decay over two months, you can be fairly confident that the ingredients are not natural.

But how on Earth can something that is so bad for us taste so good? This seeming contradiction has created a love/hate relationship between the golden sticks of yum and the American population. Recently, there have been court suits claiming that the fast food side dish is addictive and *causes* people to become fat, yet McDonald's and its tasty fried treats continue to grow in popularity. These lawsuits may seem like just a ploy to scam the system, but also bring to light the amazing addictiveness of French fries: they are ultra-condensed flavor packets and just like the super-sweeteners like neotame, produce a sensory indulgence unlike anything else.

Most people would agree that the problem isn't that these foods taste good, it's that they are so bad for us as well. Additionally, we humans are designed to enjoy things that taste like French fries, and we're not designed to avoid them like the plague. We know they're bad for us and yet, they taste so good, our will power is no match!

So with our technology, which is able to produce things like the French fry, accompanied with our seemingly weak will power, we humans are straying away from what we are naturally designed to eat. As Fogel put it, "A lush supply of food…does not necessarily mean good nutrition." Our ancestors survived by enjoying the taste of highly-caloric foods like potatoes, fat, and sugar—if they didn't, and instead enjoyed the taste of non-caloric grass or tree bark, they wouldn't have consumed enough calories to last the day, much less make it out of the Stone Age. So Nat developed a liking for sweet and fatty things in nature, but how could he have foreseen the unhealthy condensed version of those ingredients in French fries?

Our genes give us a great idea of what is healthy to eat, but when you add culture and manmade extreme foods to the equation, it's a risky proposition to trust our natural instincts. We should be able to just listen to our bodies and our genes and simply eat what tastes good, but unfortunately, the synthetic foods that taste good are tricking our taste buds into eating extremely unhealthy ingredients.

Some may ask, "Why do we continue to eat the way we do, knowing that it is the cause of our obesity and health problems?" How can we overlook such a detrimental aspect of our lives as our health? It is easy to simply say that we are designed to like the taste of doughnuts and soft drinks, and just leave it at that, but there are many reasons why we, as different cultures, eat specific things. If you are interested in why we eat specifically what we eat, we have some more exploring to do. After we have a grasp of that, we will look at how the human species would eat naturally, without the cultural and personal influences.

Cultural Influences

Our genes instruct us to seek out and eat food when our stomach shrinks, but besides that ever-present growl in our guts, there are myriad other things that are telling us to eat and, more precisely, *what* to eat. If you are a television watcher, you might have noticed the ubiquity of appetizing commercials airing—not a series of ads goes by without footage of a delicious pizza or a thick, juicy steak. Most social gatherings are accompanied by finger food and a host who wants his or her guests to leave full. If you drive in the city, the chances that you will see a billboard or a restaurant sign enticing you with mouthwatering images of cheeseburgers or French fries are quite high. We are constantly bombarded with people wanting us to eat.

Often, we acquiesce and indulge our senses in the pizza, the egg roll hors d'œuvres, or the burger because it looks so good. But those foods don't resemble natural food like fruit and vegetables that grow out in the fields, or the animal meat we're familiar with, so why do we find it appetizing? Why do pictures of a hot, greasy, ten-pound hamburger with blobs of red and yellow sauce on a puffy beige bun appeal to us? Is there an innate desire for the hamburger imbedded deep down in us—is there a hamburger gene? In other words, if Joe Schmoe had never before seen, tasted or smelled a hamburger, would a picture on a billboard make him want to eat one? To better frame this question, I'd like to alter the context a little. Imagine driving down the road and looking up to a billboard with the slogan, "How long has it been since you've tasted Heaven?" And below that slogan was a picture of a large, seasoned, grilled grasshopper. Doesn't that sound appealing? No? Well, it just might sound appealing to some native Africans when they get hungry.

Many African groups collect locusts (grasshoppers) in the morning hours before they become active, then boil them, clean them and add a bit of salt, and voila! They have a high-protein, tasty treat. Termites and caterpillars are also popular insect foods around the world. If that sounds disgusting don't be so quick to judge—we in Western culture haven't removed insects from our diet completely. A very popular Western food comes from a very unpopular insect regurgitation: honey.

Although it may sound natural to think that certain foods are disgusting and shouldn't be eaten (like termites), your feelings are most likely just something you've become accustomed to by growing up in your particular culture. Most humans have what has been dubbed neophobia (fear of something new), and despite our desire to get out and try the latest restaurant or get something different on the menu, we really only stick to the same few ingredients for all of our dishes.

Food is one of the most culturally linked products that we partake in as humans. Every culture selects a unique combination of edibles from the menu of nature, some of which tend to shock people in other cultures. Take Australia, for instance. A few years ago, I dined at a restaurant in small-town Queensland on the northeastern coast of the continent. When I ordered what I thought to be their version for shrimp, I had no idea that the little critter would come out of the kitchen with its bulging eyes staring at me! Australia is very close to America with regard to its food, but the prawns were certainly something I had to get used to.

If a relatively similar food culture like Australia's had some shocks, can you imagine what extremely different cultures would dare to eat? I found out one day when a Chinese friend of mine took me to Chicago's Chinatown district and to a common Chinese food market. My friend seemed like a normal girl with typical eating habits to me before this trip, but when I saw her indulging in the aromas and the sights of the store, I was very skeptical of her mental state. Not to gross you out, but who can think that a dried and cured pig head can look yummy? But why stop at their head, how about a little pig's feet. My experience in the Chinese market definitely gave a new meaning to the nursery rhyme *This Little Piggy*.

My favorite food oddity in the Chinese food store was the dried air bladder from a fish. My, those Chinese chefs are resourceful! Perhaps desire to utilize every animal organ in unique ways for food has something to do with the fact that the country has to feed over a billion people. I can't imagine how many people we Americans could have fed with all the dried air bladders that we've thrown away in the last couple years.

Even foods that everyone eats are served vastly differently. For instance, take the common egg. I prefer mine scrambled, with a little salt and pepper, maybe some cheese thrown on them. However, if the occasion called for it, I could find myself eating eggs poached, sunny side up, or hard-boiled. These are all normal ways of eating an egg to me. However, when I was in France, I was amused, though not necessarily appetized, by seeing a sunny side up egg sitting on top of a bowl of pasta. Similar emotions came to me when I saw that the pizza I ordered came with a bright and shiny egg right in the middle. Like a good sheltered American, I ate the egg separately.

In all my egg-eating research, nothing could have prepared me for the whopper of all egg preparations: The Chinese Thousand Year Old Egg. This masterpiece is prepared by soaking a hard-boiled egg in lime and brine until the egg white turns a gelatinous brown, and the egg yolk turns green. This is no doubt what Dr. Seuss was thinking of when he wrote *Green Eggs and Ham*. I think I'll stick with mine scrambled.

But, perhaps even our food isn't that appealing when you really take a look at it. What if I offered you a slimy white clump of live bacteria? Does it sound better when I add a gelatinous crop extract? What if I packaged it in a plastic cup with a metallic top and called it yogurt—would that appeal to you? Next on the menu: a fine specimen. A cylinder of grinded-up animal jowls (the loose, fatty flesh from the lower jaw or throat), and other parts mixed in with nitrates, which may cause health conditions, but keep foods very fresh! How does that sound? Not so appetizing? Well, when you add some mustard and relish and slip it into a warm hot dog bun at the ballpark, it sure does hit the spot!

 An Evolution Diet Essential

Culture, not genetics, dictates someone's preference for hotdogs instead of seasoned grasshoppers.

This might lead one to believe that humans can eat anything, and they can, just about. We can derive nutrition from a vast variety of foods, so why does our culture (speaking for the Americans) like hot dogs and hamburgers, but not dried air bladder or the Thousand Year Old Egg? Why can't I go to the concessions stand at the baseball stadium and order get a sunny side up egg on my pizza?

The late, great anthropologist Marvin Harris, Ph.D., who wrote many books on culture and food, said that there is an established menu in every society and the things that aren't on our menu slowly become alien to each person growing up in that environment. He said, "When you don't eat things, you end up regarding them with disgust." There's nothing innately grotesque about a bowl of pigs feet to eat, but since we grew up eating a bowl of cereal in the morning instead, the Chinese staple sounds awful.

The Chinese relied on inner Asia pastoralists for their supply of ploy animals, so they never had a need to keep cows in their villages. The result is that the food products from cows never took off in China. As Marvin Harris explains, "China never accepted dairying and the Chinese people view a glass of milk as a loathsome secretion, akin to a glass of saliva." This isn't to point out that what typical Westerners eat is disgusting, just to say that, while we could be eating Thousand Year Old Eggs and a cup of yogurt, culture directs us to eat the latter and not the former.

In addition, culture tells us what to eat as well as what to avoid. Marvin Harris explains that, "We do not come into the world entirely without taste preferences. Infants grimace and turn away from substances that taste bitter, sour, sharp, peppery, or salty." And this makes sense because most poisonous or indigestible foods have those telltale tastes. But those initial taste preferences mentioned above go away with increased exposure to healthy foods that are bitter, sour, sharp, peppery, or salty, as Marvin Harris explains:

> The Chinese love their tea scalding hot and bitter. Gauchos have their equivalent bitter drink, mate, sucked up hot from a communal cup. Americans savor their morning grapefruit chilled and cut into bite-size pieces. Spaniards squeeze lime juice on their fish. The English like their alcohol mixed with quinine water. The Germans take their meat with dollops of bitter horseradish. Sourness also abounds in world cuisines: sour milk, sour cream, sauerkraut, sourdough, sour apple. Not to mention vinegar used to pickle meat, fish, and vegetables and to mingle with oil in Italian salad dressings. Most remarkable, perhaps, is the reversal of the infantile aversion to peppery goods. In much of China, Central America,

India, Southeast Asia, and Africa, people expect to experience a tingling, burning, mouth-watering fulsomeness of fiery, hot condiments at every meal. Take away the Malabar or chili pepper, and they will rise from the table in disgust.

The food preferences that aren't culturally linked aren't just random, however. Those have a more personal origin.

Personal Influences

As a child, I remember having a vehement opposition to black pepper as a seasoning and I don't know when the conversion happened, but now, I usually don't go a dinner without putting the spicy seasoning on at least one part of the meal. If you give a baby a bit of lemon or salt, he may suffer a bit of whiplash as his face scrunches up in hilarious disagreement, but for adults, lemon and salt are two extremely popular additions to foods, and some Central Americans, who love to torture their nervous system, eat lemon with salt as a regular snack.

It seems that there is a period of time between infancy, when only certain sweet foods are palatable, and adulthood, when a liking for only certain foods has been well established, that we are pretty open for new foods. In the first few years of life, humans are usually vehemently opposed to bitter foods and generally like just sweet things, but for a few years after that, we are willing to open up our palette to everything. Erik D'Amato, in an article in *Psychology Today* said, "By age seven or eight, children learn—or are taught—what foods to consider disgusting and in what combinations palatable or even scrumptious foods become disgusting." In other words, we don't have a natural aversion to eating insects or the Thousand Year Old Egg; we are taught not to eat those things when we are young. This happens, of course, through culture, family, and friends telling us what to eat, but also special instances unique to each individual. Personal experience is another important influence on our diet.

Another way personal experience can affect ones diet is through taste aversion learning. If a woman has a deep dislike of chicken, it may have been caused by an incident in those early years. Perhaps the first few times she had chicken, it wasn't cooked thoroughly and made her sick. Incidents like this would link that sickness to that particular food for her entire life or until she decided to try el pollo loco again. Some studies show that more than 60 percent of the population has some experienced taste aversion based on a bad experience and it usually leads to irrational eating habits. A friend of mine didn't like a particular sports energy drink and he traced this aversion back to his childhood in which he only drank it when he was sick, firmly connecting the feeling of queasiness with the beverage. In my case, I became averse to cola when I was a child after I took a swig of a can in which a fly or bee had been taking a nice little cola bath. Needless to say, I didn't drink much of the stuff after that shocking experience. These experiences are pretty powerful. Alexandra Logue author of *The Psychology of Eating and Drinking* says, "Usually, a person has to get sick only once after eating a particular food in order for a taste aversion to form, and taste aversions can last an extremely long time."

First and foremost, we eat things that are available and that our culture promotes—like Pizza Hut or Papa John's with their constant barrage of advertisements—and second, we prefer items that have a good memory associated with them—like McDonald's, which makes it fun for kids to eat with Happy Meals and colorful food characters that are associated with its unnatural food.

Our personal experience makes us picky eaters, but our wealth makes us even pickier. I recently overheard a kid at a restaurant whine about how he wouldn't eat a perfectly good hamburger because he didn't like the pickle that was layered in between the lettuce and tomatoes and ketchup and mustard. Does this make any rational sense? I rather like the pickles, but with all those flavors running together, does it really make that much difference? Most likely, the complaining child was a very lucky kid who didn't know what it means to be hungry and dream of the next meal for an entire day or more.

On another dining experience, I noticed a family of four sitting next to me. I overheard their conversation and noticed that one of the kids wouldn't eat his chicken fingers because they didn't look like McDonald's Chicken McNuggets. I thought, "Maybe this kid wouldn't have such a liking for the McNuggets if he knew what 'McFrankenstein' ingredients were actually in them." Either way, he was going to make a stand and not eat his chicken fingers. Eventually I think his stomach started to question his defiance and he started to pick at them. And adults are no better—they don't have to fight with parents forcing them to eat perfectly good food, but many adults waste and complain to their waiter about seemingly ridiculous food preferences.

It may seem odd that we are so picky in a situation where there is so much good food available, but the pickiness is most likely derived from the abundance we have—we can afford to be picky and throw away perfectly good pickles and chicken fingers. This may also explain why readily available insects aren't a part of our diet and they are in parts of famished North Korea—our wealth is another reason why we don't eat what we would naturally eat. The child mentioned above who wouldn't eat his hamburger would feel fairly out of place in the Stone Age. Can you imagine a group of hunter/gatherers declining to eat a buffalo they had just captured because a pickled cucumber had touched it? Not a chance!

Of course, some food may be poisonous or otherwise unhealthy for us, and it may benefit us to avoid that food. In this respect, it's good that we are repulsed by some foods. We also have innate food standards to avoid spoiled or rancid food and we've taken that standard to an evolutionary high—a meal that might have passed for the caveman, after all, would probably make a health inspector of a local restaurant today shudder.

The healthfulness of foods in our grocery aisles is certainly one of the greatest advancements from humankind, but if someone from the pampered American culture strayed from our high standard of food, he might not be physically prepared. Imagine someone who is accustomed to America's FDA food standards visiting the great outdoors and attempting to drink from a fresh mountain stream. The bacteria present in unfiltered water can make for an unpleasant few days—digestively speaking—for the pampered Dasani drinker. Hunter/gatherers existed for millennia by drinking water out of natural rivers and streams, but our modern-day visitor wouldn't be such a happy camper. Our ancestors were used to the natural bacteria, but our bodies don't know how to fight off the little quislings. Thus, it is not only taste which people become accustomed to, but it is also the quality of food that people become accustomed to.

Regardless of the reasons why we eat what we eat, a disturbing fact remains: we have altered our menu so drastically that our natural selves—stripped of all culture and experience—would not be able to understand what we eat or how we eat currently. If we were to rely strictly on our genes' instruction for what to eat, there isn't much we would keep from our current culture-influenced menu.

What A Cultureless Human Would Eat

If we were to take away all of the culture-driven foods and get rid of the scientific mystery foods that have come along in the last few centuries, we would still find an enormous and tasty menu. We would still have all the yummy fruits, vegetables, fish, and other lean meats to consume, and if you include the scores of plants and animals that we have slowly removed from our menu over the last few hundred years, the menu becomes even more exciting and diverse. Have you ever been to a restaurant where the menu has items with a little heart icon next to it indicating a healthy food? A cultureless diet would have a little heart next to every item. If that statement makes you want to say, "That's obvious!" Then you're probably not alone.

Companies process foods to increase the food item's shelf life and make it taste better, but the more we process foods, the more they become unusable to our bodies—or worse, harmful to our bodies. Processing includes refrigerating, cooking, and of course adding preservatives and extraneous man-made ingredients, all of which change the food's makeup from something our bodies know how to digest to something that our bodies can't use.

The goal is to eat things that are tasty as well as nutritious and usable to our bodies. To some, this may mean eating only bland foods like oats or lettuce. How exciting would that be? Who wants to eat just raw vegetables and grains? You might be feeling, "If that's being healthy, then I think I'll pass." If you were to stick to a completely Stone-Age diet, the prospects may seem even worse. Not only would he have to stick to natural foods, you also would have to do without exotic foods that we have become accustomed to. Imagine a hunter/gatherer from the Paleolithic Age located in the Great Lakes region of North America. He would have to do without anything he couldn't find in his immediate vicinity: corn, berries, acorns, apples, rabbit, deer, bison, plus a

 An Evolution Diet Essential

Prehistoric man ate all types of foods, but did so according to natural abundance. They did not have a mass quantity of sweet rolls or large plates of pasta at the ready.

good deal of leafy green vegetables. He wouldn't have the pleasure of citrus fruits, large salt-water fish, peppers, cocoa, or an endless amount of tasty wonders we can find at the grocery store.

That hunter/gatherer, like the !Kung Bushmen from the Introduction, may have missed out on the culinary delights of foods from around the world, but he would be healthy because he would only be eating what he is designed to eat. Unfortunately, he probably would see eating as a chore and not the distinct pleasure that it is today. This is certainly not the idea that The Evolution Diet is trying to promote, yet it is important to know what we would eat and how we would eat it if we weren't being inundated with culture (I'll elaborate on this further in the Part Eight, Living Off the Land). From the healthy basic diet of the regional hunter/gatherer, we can apply our wealth and creativity to eating the way we were designed *and* making it just as pleasurable as it is currently.

To do this, I'm going to describe a hypothetical environment for our imaginary Stone Age subject, let's call him Nat (short for Natural Man): a person who eats without cultural influences. Nat has basically the same exact physical composition that we do today, especially regarding his digestive system, yet Nat has no culture to speak of that isn't derived directly from his natural surroundings. He builds things from the materials in his surroundings, his activities are dictated by the weather, and he eats what's around him.

Based on studies by Dr. Clark Spencer Larsen of Ohio State University and others, we know that up until recently, humans on the North American continent had a nonagricultural society which gained its nutrition from foraging and, of course, hunting. We know that before agriculture took hold in North America (around 500 A.D.), the people there were predictably less sedentary and the land was considerably less crowded. This, in turn, led to a healthier, more active population. And it wasn't as susceptible to disease as a population densely packed into a small town or city would be. Although the cities of today allow for better and quicker health treatment with the hospital, they also require that better health care because densely populated areas aid in the diffusion of sickness and disease. Luckily for us, highly advanced science has enabled us to overcome the diseases and illnesses that limited premodern city dwellers.

According to Larsen, the agriculturization of humans allowed for a constant supply of food, allowing for larger, specialized populations, but it also had drawbacks for human health. Reliance on the superfoods (e.g. wheat in Europe, rice in Asia, millet in Africa, and maize in North America) allowed less produce to feed more people but also led to poor oral health, poor bodily growth, and more disease.

As mentioned in the previous section, Larsen cites an increase in these high-carbohydrate superfoods as a cause for a shocking growth in periodontal disease around 800 A.D. in the Americas. In other words, the diet based on agriculture causes cavities. Additionally, he notes the lack of iron in these foods as a cause of smaller bodily structures over the same time period. Finally, he states that the sedentary lifestyle of the large populations that depended on farming was "conducive to the maintenance and spread of infectious disease."

So, what did Nat eat if he didn't have the food pyramid to guide him? How could prehistoric man have been so healthy as to make it out there in the wilderness, without modern medicine or health care? And how could he have been so successful? Even with his highly stressful life, the average Paleolithic man lived up to 40 years of age in the Mesolithic period (10,000 B.C. to 6,000 B.C.), well beyond childbearing age.

It is probable that humans before agriculturization ate all types of food, including the superfoods that weren't toxic (like rice and maize), but did so in a less structured, less methodical way than we do today. More importantly, they ate it according to the natural abundance. They did not have a mass quantity of concentrated high fructose corn syrup or large rice dishes readily available. What they did have was mass quantities of green leafy vegetables and to a lesser extent, denser vegetables like carrots and fruits like apples. Also fairly plentiful were nuts (like the !Kung favorite mongongo) and berries. Of course, the modern staples like corn were also available to some extent.

The pre-modern man (before agriculturization) would constantly be eating these abundant natural foods to ward off their hunger. Some hunter/gatherers, like the Iroquois of North America, were even adept at creating treats like today's Cracker Jacks by making maple syrup and drizzling it over popcorn. But, unlike modern humans who have the ability to reach into a bag of Cracker Jacks and pull out a handful the sugary snack, it would take some time and effort to create the Iroquois version and the pre-modern version wouldn't have artificial ingredients like corn syrup, refined sugar, vegetable oil, salt, or soy lecithin. The all-natural version was just as tasty, but much healthier.

Outside of the Iroquois caramel corn, most of the gathered

food Natural Man ate (e.g. berries) required no preparation. He would pick at the berry bush or flower patch for a long period of time, slowly ingesting what nowadays we would eat in one large super-sized bite. This practice of constantly eating, but eating slowly does two things: it moderates the intake of food, thus stabilizing the intake of energy through the digestive system, and also keeps the eater's metabolism at a constant rate. We will discuss these two characteristics of the diet in the next chapter, but keep this in mind: for the most part, Nat wanted to keep eating constantly. This is why those of us who are obese can legitimately blame their condition on their genes. We are designed to put food in our mouths constantly; the major divergence between our ancestors and us is that Nat ate healthy fibrous foods constantly, whereas today we eat unhealthy and calorically-dense foods constantly.

We are designed to eat mainly two types of foods — energy and protein. The default provision of choice was plant food, which was defenseless (for the most part) and found everywhere. When Nat and his friends got enough energy from their foraging menu, they would have sought a more substantially nutritious food by hunting, which entailed running after large game and working to trap it or kill it. But today, unless you are a politician looking for publicity before a big election, you probably don't claim to be a hunter. That's okay — any exercise is a good substitute for Nat's hunting. To be completely healthy and as efficient as we can be as a species, we must not settle on the scant protein of nuts and plants, but rather, we must hunt (to put it into primitive terms) the extremely rich foods, which animals are. And, with the energy needs taken care of from his constant foraging of carbohydrates throughout the day, Nat would have been able to use the proteins he ate after the hunt to help build and repair his body. Having a sufficient amount of protein is important, especially for those who exercise heavily, as we will see in the next section.

The hunter/gatherer society, which had just successfully hunted a large animal would be able to then gorge on this immediately abundant food source. And it is important that they do so to avoid the bacteria — Prehistoric man could not rely on refrigeration or cooking to retard or kill the bacteria on their leftovers. Although cooking is used to kill off the bacteria, which find themselves attracted to meat, humans can safely digest raw meat if eaten within a reasonable time period (one to two days). Our stomach is a powerful incinerator, which can take in just about any food or bacteria without ill effect, but leaving meat in the open for too long can make the food inedible, even for our stomachs.

When dense protein is present in the stomach, HCl is released at a faster rate and the acidity is increased in the stomach to below pH 2. This high acidity enables the digestion of the protein and the killing of the bacteria. If there is a large amount of dense carbohydrates in the stomach at the same time, the pH is raised and acidity lowered, making it more difficult for the stomach to digest the protein properly. The result is putrefaction of the meat and fermentation of the carbohydrates. This process creates a great deal of gas and makes it more difficult for the body to take in the needed nutrition. It might not be that beans are the "magical fruit," and the "more you eat them, the more you toot." Rather, it may just be that people eat beans with the wrong foods (e.g. beef) and thus, our body doesn't react kindly to them.

You can see that even though the actual foods Nat ate were fairly close to what we eat today in terms of basic components, he had a vastly different eating style than we do. Nat and his community ate one thing, like berries, for an extended amount of time and then moved on to a lettuce patch, which he then consumed for an extended amount of time. They gained variety through time, not all at once, as in the modern balanced meal. They focused on one type of naturally occurring fruit or vegetable, maybe a couple at a time, and then moved on to a different location and also a different plant. After they were done with the surrounding plants, they hunted, and then gorged on meat until they were full. They did not have the food pyramid diet, promoting every food group in each meal; in fact, the idea of a modern meal is completely lost with Nat and his family. While they did get all of their vitamins and minerals, they did so in a less uniform manner.

Separating one's food sources is called appropriating one's diet and we can do it without adverse effects because many of the vitamins we need (the fat-soluble vitamins A, D, E, and K) are stored in our body for long periods of time. The water-soluble vitamins (B-complex and C), however, are not stored and must be replenished daily.

Apart from vitamin intake, Nat's style of spacing out his intake of different foods optimized his body's ability to focus on certain things and change the physiological reaction in his stomach to suit the content. This method of eating, which will be described further in Part Four, extracts the most nutrition from the food one takes in as well as keeps one's metabolism going on a fairly consistent path, one that our bodies are designed for.

Part Four
The Body's Physiology
(What Makes Us Go)

"The toughest part of a diet isn't watching what you eat. It's watching what other people eat."

-Dieter

Q: If you split a can of diet cola with one calorie into two glasses, which glass gets the calorie?

Bacon, sausage, eggs, hamburgers, cheese—it's all okay to eat as long as it's protein! That's what some fad diet promoters may tell you. They'll tell you that just need to focus on just one type of macronutrient (e.g. protein) to be completely healthy. Others may recommend that you scrutinize every facet of your diet down to the exact calorie level of everything you put into your body. I believe the former version of a diet is too simplified and the latter version is far too complex. When it comes down to it, there isn't a lone miracle cure that will make you healthy and, likewise, it's not necessary for us to count every calorie and spend hours looking on the nutrition information panels at the grocery store to ensure the right percentage of protein, carbohydrate, and fat content of our food.

The reality is that there are 44 essential ingredients that we need to survive and those can be broken down into seven categories: amino acids, fatty acids, vitamins, minerals, carbohydrates, and water. Though some nutrients are more important than others, without any one of those basic ingredients, we would cease to work as a living organism—everything else we need we can create ourselves. The essentials are listed as follows:

Amino Acids

- Histidine
- Isoleucine
- Lysine
- Leucine
- Methionine
- Phenylalanine
- Threonine
- Tryptophan
- Valine
- Arginine

Fatty Acids

- Linolenic acid (the shortest chain omega-3 fatty acid)
- Linoleic acid (the shortest chain omega-6 fatty acid)

Vitamins

- Biotin (vitamin B7, vitamin H)
- Choline (vitamin Bp)
- Folate (folic acid, vitamin B9, vitamin M)
- Niacin (vitamin B3, vitamin P, vitamin PP)

- Pantothenic acid (vitamin B5)
- Riboflavin (vitamin B2, vitamin G)
- Thiamine (vitamin B1)
- Vitamin A (retinol)
- Vitamin B6 (pyridoxine, pyridoxamine, or pyridoxal)
- Vitamin B12 (cobalamin)
- Vitamin C (ascorbic acid)
- Vitamin D (Cholecalciferol, Ergocalciferol, Calcitriol)
- Vitamin E (tocopherol)
- Vitamin K (naphthoquinoids)

Minerals
- Calcium (Ca)
- Chloride (Cl-)
- Cobalt (Co)
- Copper (Cu)
- Iodine (I)
- Iron (Fe)
- Magnesium (Mg)
- Manganese (Mn)
- Molybdenum (Mo)
- Phosphorus (P)
- Potassium (K)
- Selenium (Se)
- Sodium (Na)
- Sulfur (S)
- Zinc (Zn)

Fatty acids are important for formation of healthy cell structures and the proper functioning of the brain and nervous system. Amino acids are the building materials we need to create proteins and much of the physical matter in our bodies—without them, we would be barely anything but water and fat. Vitamins and minerals are the life process facilitators that individually do a variety of beneficial services for us humans such as protect against free radicals (antioxidants), help you digest certain things like calcium, and help in every basic life function, like burning energy.

While all of the above ingredients are vital, there is nothing more important to our health than water. Water, which will be emphasized in Part Ten, makes up over 60 percent of our entire body weight and is impossible to live without. A human can live weeks without any food energy, but only a couple days without taking in any water. We're lucky that water can be found in almost everything we eat. One doesn't have to drink half their body weight in water each day to stay healthy because H_2O is in the fruits and vegetables and to a lesser extent meats and nuts that we eat all the time. That doesn't mean that one shouldn't drink as much water as is reasonable. A sufficient amount of water is vital to everything from warding off headaches to keeping skin healthy.

All of the aforementioned nutrients are staples in a healthy diet and all dietitians and nutritionists would agree that you should maintain a diet with plenty of amino acids, vitamins, minerals, and water. The main choice that we have with regard to our diets, and the main point of contention in nutrition books, is what form of energy we consume. Since we can get necessary energy in four very distinct ways, there has been much debate over what the best way to attain our energy is, as anyone who has been on an extremely low-carb diet or a lettuce diet can attest. The four forms of edible energy are carbohydrates, proteins, fats, and alcohols. All have unique attributes that make them beneficial or deleterious and, as with most things we can ingest, there is a limit to how much one should be eating of each. I will discuss each energy type in thrilling detail and explain the pros and cons for each one with respect to diet in general and touch on how each fits into The Evolution Diet: All-Natural and Allergy Free.

Carb Is Not A Four Letter Word

With recent diet books on the market such as the Atkins plan, many people have gained an extreme aversion to the friendly little molecules of carbon and water (hydrogen and oxygen = hydrate). Some people have gone so far as to ban the energy type from their diet, entirely. Others have taken measures so drastic to limit their carbohydrate intake that it seems like just eating less altogether would be easier and less painful than adhering to such a strict gimmicky diet to lose weight. It appears our culture has gotten a little out of hand: commercials promoting a beer with 1 gram of carbs fewer than a competitor's; orders at a restaurant like, "Could I have the burger meal deal, no bun, no tomato, hold the fries, but could I get a little cup of the grease you fry them in?" Some people endure endless supermarket trips with constant perusing of the ingredients panels looking for the zero-carb food that actually tastes good. I even know people who have had nightmares little carbs chasing after them.

The Evolution Diet is here to stop the madness! Carbohydrates are not the end of the world. In fact, they are quite necessary for optimal health. Researchers at the MedStar Research Institute in Washington, D.C. have found that, despite the recent negative connotation carbohydrates have with regard to weight gain; increasing healthy carbs (not simple sugars) can be good for most people. Barbara Howard, at the Institute said, "Our study shows that increasing carbohydrates as we did it, with an emphasis on vegetables and fruits and nuts, in fact does not promote weight gain." So put the bacon down, you can eat carbohydrates again! Diets such as the Zone and Atkins push the unending benefits of protein as an energy source and blame all health problems today on carbohydrates. Those methods of eating may help you lose weight — at least for a few weeks — but they will be contrary to what your body is designed for and cause a significant amount of stress on the inner workings of your body.

What's In A Carb?

Carbohydrate is the general term for an extremely versatile type of molecule. There are two main types of carbohydrates that we digest: simple sugars and complex carbohydrates. There is a very important difference between the two because the body treats them extremely differently. Although they are both made of the same basic components, they are composed in very different ways. The basic chemical formula for a carbohydrate looks like this: $C_6H_{12}O_6$. This is the simplest form of a carbohydrate called glucose.

Glucose is the preferred energy source used by all the cells in our bodies. When we intake other types of sugars, they are broken down into glucose so that the cells can use it. Glucose is so simple, that there is absolutely NO digestion needed to make the substance useable by our cells. If you were to sip a yummy glass of fresh glucose juice, the molecules would flow directly from your digestive tract into your bloodstream, hence another name for glucose: blood sugar.

The fact that it can enter our bloodstream so quickly without any middleman is a benefit, in that it can give us a boost of energy when we need it, but glucose can also be a hazard. If you need

Tips On Energy Sources

• A calorie is the energy it takes to heat 1 gram of water by 1 degree Celsius.

• What people call a calorie everyday is actually a kilocalorie, or 1000 calories defined above.

• A gram of carbohydrate has 4 calories, a gram of protein has 4 calories, a gram of alcohol has 7 calories, and a gram of fat contains 9 calories.

• 3,500 calories is equivalent to 1 pound of fat.

• Although most nutrition labels cite a 2,000 calorie diet, the actual recommended intake for an average active person is 2,500 calories per day.

• It takes the human body different amounts of time to get to the energy contained within different food types.

that instant kick, a frothy glucose beverage is just what the doctor ordered, but if you're not in any need of energy, this boost might make you irritable, tense, or stressed. Our bodies have their way of moderating any spike in energy like one you'd get from chugging that cup o' glucose, but the effects are still potent, especially when one ingests pure glucose (or simple sugars).

You might say, "But, I've never ordered a frothy glucose shake before." Perhaps you haven't ordered it by name, but every time you open a soda can you're basically drinking glucose straight. You can find glucose in honey, grape juice, and corn from which we can derive a form of glucose called cornstarch. Other fruits have a similar molecule in them called fructose, which has the same chemical makeup as glucose, but the atoms are in slightly different places. Galactose is another one-celled sugar, or monosaccharide, but is only found naturally connected with glucose. Fructose and galactose can also take rides through our bloodstream because they are so simple — more complex molecules need a little bit of work before the body can use them directly.

Glucose Molecule ($C_6H_{12}O_6$)

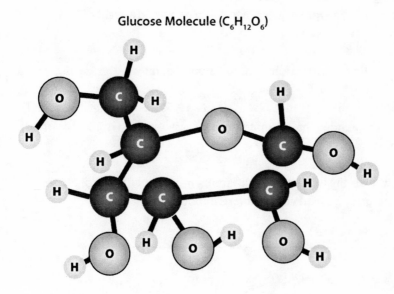

Interestingly enough, glucose is about half as sweet as table sugar, which is a disaccharide that contains a glucose molecule and a fructose molecule. Disaccharides (meaning contains two monosaccharide molecules) are just a bit more complicated than the single molecule sugars, but are broken down very easily in our digestive tract, as well. Common disaccharides are sucrose (table sugar), lactose (the sugar in milk), and maltose (the sugar in, you guessed it, malt).

Sugar definitely gets around, and has many pseudonyms. If you want a laugh sometime, look on the ingredients of a candy bar and count the number of ingredients which are really different names for the same thing: sugar. A Snicker's bar lists that same substance (sugar) five times as different ingredients. Pop Tarts list that same ingredient nine times! Manufacturers can disguise the name sugar as any of the following: corn syrup, dextrose, lactose, galactose, fructose, glucose, high-fructose corn syrup (HFCS), honey, invert sugar, levulose, molasses, or sucrose. Sometimes, candies actually use the word 'sugar' too.

These all taste sweet, which is an immediate indication of their potency. These sugars are ready to get the body going, and fast! If you eat a large amount of a simple sugar, you should feel the effects immediately. You should feel more awake, more alert, and you should have more strength and energy. This is the imme-diate result, though it's not sustained — after a spike in blood sugar, a non-diabetic will get a spike in insulin, usually over-compensat-ing for the sugar and causing opposite results. All of us have, at some point, experienced the lull after a sugar high. Perhaps you've had one too many soda pops or you've decimated your trick or treat bag and you've been wired and bouncing off walls for the last half hour, when all of the sudden, you start to come down. This is your body catching up with you. The sugar high that you just had was a result of mass quantities of glucose being released into the bloodstream — much more than was needed for normal operation. The average human body needs about two teaspoons of glucose to do what it needs to do at any given time and a lot of that comes from the more complex energy sources that you've been digesting for the last few hours. When you take in foods with sugar as the number one ingredient, you're most likely taking in three to four times as much glucose as you need. If you drink a typical soda pop, you're putting in three tablespoons of sugar, or four and a half times the needed amount, in your body.

There are a few organs that are involved in controlling your blood sugar level, your hypothalamus and your pituitary glands in your brain, and the pancreas in your abdomen. There are little peanut-like formations of cells spread out on the pancreas called the Islets of Langerhans. This is the vital organ that gives us energy stability through the ever-important insulin.

Insulin controls the amount of blood sugar in your blood, and if your body is only used to a little glucose coming in at a time, as is the case for most people, it's going to take a while for those little peanuts to crank out the needed insulin to regulate the blood sugar after a influx of blood glucose. Insulin feeds the glucose to the cells (sugar high), and when the cells have had all they can handle, the same remarkable hormone, insulin, brings all the excess glucose in the blood to the liver to convert it to a complex carbohydrate (and you feel the sugar low). If you took in too much sugar for even that process to handle, the excess glucose is converted into fat. There is an appropriate amount of sugar the body should intake and as we will see later.

With such an amazing amount of stress caused by glucose, it's hard to imagine that it's good for you at all, but it is extremely important. While there are three monosaccharides that can flow through the bloodstream, glucose is the preferred energy source of the brain, outside of starvation. Maintaining your glucose level is important, not only for energy, but also mental wellbeing. Fortunately, you can eat complex carbohydrates to receive the glucose you need and you can avoid the drastic sugar highs and lows that simple sugars cause.

Sugar High

We know that our body tries to maintain a constant blood sugar level and the ups and glucose contribute to a high level of stress by our internal organs. When this stress becomes too much for the body to handle, bad things can happen. Type II Diabetes is one of those bad things. When there is a consistent pattern of excess caloric intake (All-U-Can-Eat at Joe's Diner) with a deficient caloric expenditure (sitting on the couch instead of exercising), the body fights against itself. First, it starts to ignore that ever-important hormone insulin. With habitual overeating, the body stops producing insulin all together, and when the body's natural infrastructure that deals with maintaining blood sugar levels is tampered with or damaged, one has to maintain those levels manually. This is why diabetes patients must inject themselves with insulin on a regular basis. If want to go easy on needles in the future, it might be a good idea to go easy on the sugar now.

This diabetic self-maintenance of blood sugar levels can be done safely and effectively, but often involves a dramatic shift in one's lifestyle and behavior. If a diabetic doesn't moderate their blood sugar, the results can be blindness and a lower life expectancy. There are other less critical symptoms; webMD lists some interesting symptoms as the following: Feeling dizzy, tingling, blurred or distorted vision or seeing flashes of light; seeing large, floating red or black spots; or seeing large areas that look like floating hair, cotton fibers, or spider webs. Outside of Allman Brothers' concertgoers in the '70s, I don't think anyone would want to experience symptoms like these; diabetes is a serious illness and must be treated as such.

When something as important as insulin is not being made by your body, that means that your body is not working for you any more. The rise in diabetes in Western culture can be attributed to people's diets not conforming to the way we were designed to eat. The Evolution Diet: All-Natural and Allergy Free aids your body and helps its natural processes to regulate insulin and to alleviate the stress caused by unnatural eating habits.

One of the key factors in preventing diabetes is eating for your lifestyle. One should only sugary foods if one is expending a lot of energy. That makes perfect sense, right: you should take in what you expend. The only reason you need to fill your system with a mouthful of sugar is when you're running or kayaking, or playing high-stakes dodge ball. Even then, the sugar you consume should be natural in origin, not the artificial chemicals found in sodas. Grapes, oranges, or carrots are great high-sugar foods that are natural and healthy.

You may notice that if you do eat a candy bar or drink a glass of orange juice, and you're not exercising, you may feel energetic, wired, or even anxious or irritable. These are natural reactions to a bulk of sugar entering your bloodstream. It is your body telling you to use that energy and go exercise.

The Yale Guide to Children's Nutrition explains that the body's reaction to high sugar foods is cause for some adverse effects if we aren't eating for any purpose other than energy. If one eats an excess of sugar and doesn't use it, there could be problems:

> ...when a child eats a sweet food, such as a candy bar or
> a can of soda, the glucose level of the blood rises rapidly. In
> response, the pancreas secretes a large amount of insulin to
> keep blood glucose levels from rising too high. This large
> insulin response in turn tends to make the blood sugar fall
> to levels that are too low 3 to 5 hours after the candy bar

or can of soda has been consumed. This tendency of blood glucose levels to fall may then lead to an adrenaline surge, which in turn can cause nervousness and irritability... The same roller-coaster ride of glucose and hormone levels is not experienced after eating complex carbohydrates ...because the digestion and absorption processes are much slower.

The last part of this is extremely important, "The same roller-coaster ride of glucose and hormone levels is not experienced after eating complex carbohydrates..." (e.g. whole-wheat breads, salads, vegetables, whole-grain rice, nuts and other high-fiber foods). Although these foods have very high amounts of carbohydrates, the amount of sugar is relatively low so it is more difficult to digest and get to the energy. It takes an extremely more complex process to get to the basic glucose molecules in broccoli or even bread than a soda pop.

When you intake high-sugar foods your body takes in glucose at a rate of 30 calories per minute, while a complex carbohydrate gives you just 2 calories per minute. That's a whopping 15 times the ingestion rate. If you were to eat the same amount of calories in bread as in a glass of grape juice, you would notice no sugar spike with the bread and a dramatic spike in blood sugar levels with the juice.

Something you may have heard a great deal about recently is the glycemic index (GI) of a particular food. GI is the rate that a given food increases one's blood sugar. This index is extremely questionable in its clinical legitimacy, but the concept is worth noting. Some foods affect your body with increased blood sugar more than others. Within the category of fruits, apples have a low GI (38), while dates have a high GI (103). Typically, the low glycemic foods are great for constant eating throughout the day in low quantities and the high glycemic foods are suitable only before and during exercise.

Note that while the glycemic index may be telling of the potency of each particular food, it is also important to factor in another trendy term: the glycemic load. While the glycemic index is measured by judging the equal weights of foods (50 grams of carbohydrate from apples compared with 50 grams of carbohydrate from dates to arrive at the figures listed above), it would be a lot more difficult to eat fifty grams of apples, since they are relatively light. This is important when you see something like the glycemic index of carrots (131). When compared with pasta, which has a GI of 71, carrots seem very bad for you, but one would have to eat a pound and a half of carrots to eat the 50 grams necessary to get to that 131 GI. Glycemic load takes portion size into account, thus the GL of carrots is 3.5 and the GL of pasta is 23.5. Note that the scale between glycemic index and glycemic load are different (GL 23.5 is high, whereas GI 131 is high).

Another thing to keep in mind when you look at the glycemic index of foods is the control substance used to achieve the GI. There are two common comparisons: glucose at GI 100, and a slice of white bread at GI 100. These two different controls give extremely different variations of GI, although they are always proportional. A baked potato has a glycemic index of 85 compared to pure glucose, but a whopping 121 compared to white bread. Brown rice is GI 55 compared to glucose and GI 79 compared to white bread. If you were to compare the incompatible figures of brown rice and a baked potato, you might think that they are very similar (85 to 79), but in reality their glycemic effect is vastly different, according to these studies.

Besides its usefulness, there are some obvious flaws with the index. If you compare breakfast cereals, for instance, you will find that sugarless Corn Flakes has a relatively high GI of 80, while a sugary cousin, Frosted Flakes has a GI of 50. Pretzels are also pretty high with a GI of 83, but a snickers bar is a healthy GI 41. If this makes you scratch your head about the glycemic index, you're not alone. The American Diabetes Association has not endorsed the index, citing high amounts of doubt in its clinical utility. The ADA says that priority should be given to amount, rather than the source of carbohydrate.

In general, if you want to determine how a particular food is going to affect your blood sugar, listen to your taste buds. A food that is dense and tastes sweet is going to spike your blood sugar.

We Are Made of Protein

That title is almost correct. We're actually only 20 percent protein, another 60 percent water, and the rest is minerals (e.g. calcium in your bones). A person without protein however, would look a lot like one of the scary skeleton pirates from Pirates of the Caribbean. Suffice it to say that a healthy diet is protein wealthy. Protein is so nutritious that we humans can pretty much get most of what we need from high-protein foods—they contain all we need to make energy, promote growth, and aid in the digestion of minerals. The question then becomes, why do we need to eat anything else?

The truth of the matter is that while protein is very versatile, it's extremely stressful on our bodies to use amino acids (the constituent compounds of protein) for anything but building blocks. In fact, for the body to use proteins as energy, a process called protein metabolism, the body must imitate its reaction to an extremely stressful situation—say, running away from a hungry bear. In a stressful situation like that, fat is mobilized from storage (converted to sugars), blood sugar increases, blood pressure increases, minerals are drawn from the blood, and proteins are pulled from the thymus and the lymph glands are turned into sugars immediately.

When there is little availability of carbohydrates, the body turns to protein metabolism for energy. The first step is the breakdown of proteins into smaller amino acids and the injection of these molecules into the blood stream, increasing blood pressure. While amino acid content in the blood is high, the body releases two opposing hormones, insulin and glucagon. Insulin lowers the blood sugar level, while glucagon raises it. These two hormones are usually released at different times to regulate blood sugar, but during protein metabolism, they are both needed to ensure the process. This is safe in people who aren't diabetic, but is considerably more stressful to just get energy from carbohydrates.

The second step of protein metabolism is the breakdown of the amino acids into what are basically a carbohydrate structure and a nitrogen component. This nitrogen unit is great when paired with a carbon unit, but is pretty useless alone, and in fact, it's dangerous at certain levels. The nitrogen unit pulled from the amino acid (usually ammonia) is removed from the blood stream through the kidneys. After all this, the near-carbohydrate unit, called a carbon skeleton, can then be broken down and used for energy.

If this process seems like a lot of stress to get a couple of calories of energy, you're right. If there was an ample amount of carbohydrates in one's diet, the eater would be able to use the carbohydrates for energy and use proteins for their natural purpose: cell building. This is why diets with sufficient carbohydrates have been proven to provide more sustainable energy for exercise and general liveliness. In addition, an appropriate level of carbohydrates in the diet will reduce blood pressure and the poisonous nitrogen content in the body, reducing unnecessary stress on the liver and kidneys.

Having stated the danger of consuming solely proteins, it is necessary to note that the body can't survive on just carbohydrates. The body needs protein and most people today are deficient in this aspect of a complete diet.

Amino Acid Molecule ($C_3H_4O_2NK_3$)
Amino Acids are one component of a protein molecule

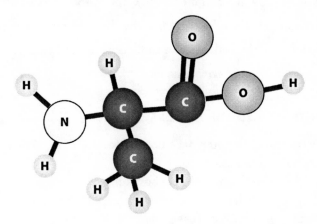

Humans need amino acids— taurine, glucoronolactone, and tryptophan to name a few of the more popular ones—to support life. The body distinguishes these amino acids into two categories: essential and nonessential. We can make the nonessential amino acids from other things in our bodies, but we cannot create the essential amino acids ourselves, so we must get them from the food we take in.

The Recommended Daily Allowance of protein is 0.36 grams per pound of body weight. A person who weighs 160 pounds would need to consume 57.6 grams of protein a day. A small can of tuna has 33 grams, so you can see that it doesn't take much high-protein food to achieve the recommended amount. When you exercise, however, your body requires more protein to rebuild the muscle tissue you've just damaged and build more. Conversely if one doesn't exercise, one doesn't need as much protein.

Regardless of the amount of protein in one's diet, it is very important for the digestion of vital amino acids that you eat the protein separately from mass amounts of carbohydrates. This concept was first promoted by The Evolution Diet and also incidentally flies in the face of conventional knowledge spurred on by the promotion of the balanced meal. We've been told that a balanced meal is the only way to be truly healthy, but, as you'll see, eating protein and carbohydrates at the same time is not healthy, and in fact leads to unwanted consequences.

 An Evolution Diet Essential

If there is an ample amount of carbohydrates in your diet, you can use those for energy, and use proteins for what they are best at: cell building. If you have no carbohydrates in your system, your body will use protein for energy in a stressful process.

From the paper *Gastrointestinal Hormones and Food Intake* by April Strader, PhD. and Stephen Woods, PhD., and others, we already know that the stomach releases specific hormones depending on the content of the eater's meal, but how exactly does different food change digestion? When protein is taken into the stomach, the hormone gastrin signals the release of HCl, which lowers the pH level in the stomach to below pH 2. The high level of HCl is important because the stomach also releases the protease pepsin in order to break down the chicken burrito or the seared ahi in our guts, but pepsin only works with sufficient HCl. Without high acidity, pepsin can't do its job and the protein moves along the digestive tract undigested and unusable by our bodies. The pH level in the next stage of digestion, the small intestine, is far more neutral (around 6.5), and thus, pepsin cannot operate.

Amylase is the enzyme that breaks down carbohydrates, but it can only be active in neutral pH environments like the mouth or the small intestine. If carbohydrates are present in the stomach, they will act to increase the pH of the stomach (lower the acidity) and reduce the effectiveness of pepsin. In this way, carbohydrates inhibit the proper digestion of protein in the stomach by lowering the overall acidity. Because of this, it is important to separate the ingestion of mainly protein and mainly carbohydrate foods for optimal enzyme production and performance. This goes straight to the heart of the second principle of The Evolution Diet, which is: Appropriate your diet.

If you choose to follow the concept of a balanced meal, which often combines a high-protein food like beef with a high-carb food like mashed potatoes, the result is incomplete digestion, which can present itself in various unpleasant and often smelly ways. Everyone who has been diagnosed with lactose intolerance can attest to the pains and trouble that poor digestion causes. Lactose intolerant people can't digest the sugar in milk products and if they drink milk or a tall milkshake, the consequences can be explosive—literally. Gas is the result of consuming something we don't digest, whether it's because our bodies don't produce the necessary enzyme (lactase in the case of lactose intolerance) or because our diet inhibits the enzymes we have (pepsin in the case of a balanced-meal eater).

Proper digestion is extremely important to overall health and maximizing your enzyme productivity is vital to your digestion, as the recent interest in enzyme therapy has shown. A study from the National Center for Health Statistics revealed that more than 60 million Americans suffer from some form of digestive disorder, many of which result in deadly diseases like cancer. The conditions range from constipation and gallstones to ulcers and acid reflux disease and can show up in symptoms like chronic fatigue, premature aging, arthritis, poor skin and hair quality, toxicity, and allergies. So many Americans are suffering from digestive problems because too many Americans are not appropriating their diets like they were designed to do.

And it makes sense. The natural hunter/gatherer (Nat) didn't eat a balanced meal. He would instead pick at a food—most likely a high-fiber carbohydrate—while "gathering" in a certain area for an extended period of time. Then, he would hunt an animal and eat his fill of the high-protein meat. While Nat's feasting on his recently captured large game, though, he wouldn't be wondering what mashed potatoes would taste like accompany the meat—the potatoes would be available to him long after the nutritious meat would. In other words, Nat wouldn't be eating fruits and vegetables with his woolly mammoth meal.

Since Nat's hunting usually took place while it was light out but probably after the hottest time of day (usually around 3 o'clock), it is assumed that the gorging of the animal occurred in the evening, preceding sleep. And it just so happens that a meal of this type (large and high-protein) is ideal before sleep due to a number of factors. When someone takes in a massive meal, the body concentrates a higher amount of energy to the digestion of the meal in thermogenesis, which makes the eater more tired. Although many specialists today ask their patients not to eat a large meal before sleeping, doing so is actually natural protocol, especially if the meal is high in protein. Just think of how sleepy you get at your desk after eating a large lunch.

In addition to the effects of a large meal on one's energy level, there is another advantage that the hunter's evening feast has over the balanced meal. Anyone who has eaten too much turkey during Thanksgiving will attest to the sleep-conducive powers of the turkey amino acid, tryptophan. This essential amino acid plays an important role in creating niacin, which, in turn, helps produce the sleep aid serotonin. But, it's not just turkey that has this snooze stuff. Cheese, milk, tofu, seafood, beef, poultry, eggs, and nuts also have a healthy amount of tryptophan.

In fact, since tryptophan is an amino acid, it can be found in high amounts in most high-protein foods, but not in high-energy foods. With the notable exception of bananas, very few high-sugar foods have a lot of the sleep-inducer. Based on our reaction to protein, most notably tryptophan, it's clear that our bodies were designed to eat the foods listed above in high quantities before rest, while the high sugar/carbohydrate foods should be limited before sleep. *The Evolution Diet: All-Natural and Allergy Free* recommends that you to eat protein at the end of the day, preferably after exercise, and before sleep in order to aid in that process.

Tryptophan takes about an hour to reach the brain after consumption and it works best on an empty stomach, so eat your protein appropriately when planning your sleep schedule. Also, the earlier you eat at night, the sooner you will be hungry the next morning. If you have trouble sleeping, it may be caused by hunger, so the later the meal, the less likely you will be hungry throughout the night.

With Friends Like Fats, Who Needs Enemies?

Just like protein, we need fats to lead a healthy life, so in a way, fats are our friends. There are two major functions (besides energy storage) that fat has: vitamin absorption and bodily support.

Although the most commonly known roll of fat is to store energy so that we may go days without food, another integral roll for the food is the digestion of vitamins. There are thirteen vitamins essential for humans and four of those require fat to be present to be used by the body. These fat-soluble vitamins protect against things like night blindness, rickets, anemia, and poor blood clotting.

Another vital role of fat is on the cellular level. Just like certain amino acids from protein, we need certain fatty acids from fats that we can't create ourselves. These essential fatty acids support the cardiovascular, reproductive, immune, and nervous systems. They come in two forms that you may hear in commercial advertisements and news reports: omega-3 and omega-6 fatty acids. Along with the nonessential fatty acid omega-9, these are the good fats as long as the consumption ratio is balanced (recent studies show that a 3-parts omega-6 to 1-part omega-3 ratio is ideal but that most Americans take in an imbalanced 20 to 1 ratio). You can find omega-3 essential fatty acids in foods as diverse as flax seeds, salmon, peppermint leaves, soybeans, and kale, whereas omega-6 fatty acids are mainly found in vegetable oils and eggs.

It is important to note that, with regard to energy, fats are fairly easy to burn. Since we store all of our excess energy as fats, though, our bodies see fat as excess energy and without increased exercise, the fat will remain as fat and not be turned into energy.

There are two main types of fats, which represent what some clever people have termed the good fats and the bad fats: unsaturated and saturated. Unsaturated fats are the more beneficial types and the essential fatty acids are in this category. These fats are liquid at room temperature and come from plant sources, most commonly olives, peanuts, and soybeans (though we'll see in the next part that peanuts and soybeans should be avoided for other reasons). Saturated fats are those that are solid at room temperature and these are the bad fats with very little benefits. These fats tend to raise cholesterol levels more than the ingestion of cholesterol itself and usually come from animal sources and include lard.

Some oils, though they are liquid at room temperature, are not 100 percent unsaturated. Check the nutritional information and ingredients to get the content of the oils before you buy them. If you have some oils with saturated fat content, you can separate the two by placing the oil in the refrigerator. After a couple hours, the saturated fats will separate and become solid.

Fat Molecule ((CH_2)$_2$$CH_3$($COOH$)$_3$)
Fat is also known as a triglyceride

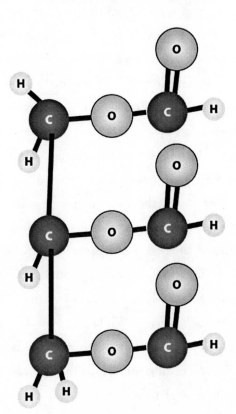

There is one type of man-made fat that everyone should be particularly aware of and should make a concerted effort to avoid. That fat is hydrogenated or partially-hydrogenated oil. As mentioned before, oil is a type of unsaturated fat, which can be healthy in moderation. Oil from vegetables such as olive oil, which is a mono-unsaturated fat, can help reduce blood cholesterol levels and help reduce the risk of coronary disease. However, food production companies started altering natural oils in the beginning of the 20th century and what they created was extremely unhealthy.

By heating natural oils in the presence of a metal catalyst and hydrogen, liquid oils turn solid. The benefit of this was its ability to replace more costly natural solid fats like lard. The production and use of these hydrogenated oils, or trans fats, increased until the 1960s and health *benefits* were even attributed to them. Unfortunately, they are extremely bad for us and have a uniquely adverse affect on blood lipid levels and lead to coronary disease.

Many countries in Europe have planned the banning of all trans fats in food, and the US Food and Drug Administration has seen enough evidence to require food producers to list the fats on the nutrition labels. Until they do this, you can identify unhealthy foods by looking for "hydrogenated" or "partially-hydrogenated oil" in the ingredients. Avoid them as much as possible.

One thing to be aware of regarding trans-fats is a regulation on the packaging of foods with partially hydrogenated oils. Manufacturers are allowed to claim their product has, "No Trans-Fats!" or, "0 grams of Trans-Fats!" if it has less than 0.5 grams of the artificial filler in each serving. While that may seem reasonable if a serving size is a cup or two, when a serving size is around two tablespoons as it is with peanut butter, the ratio increases. We recommend that you look at the list of ingredients instead of relying on product advertisements.

Part Five
Allergens and Toxins
(What Slows Us Down)

"What is food to one man may be fierce poison to others."

-Lucretius

"In general, mankind, since the improvement of cookery, eats twice as much as nature requires"

-Benjamin Franklin

Friends of mine were out enjoying a happy hour at a local brewery when one friend, Kim, asked another what he was eating because it looked mighty tasty. He replied that it was a quesadilla with cheese, black beans, and chicken and that it was as good as it looked. In the grand scheme of things, the quesadilla wasn't the worst thing to eat—it was made with all-natural ingredients (albeit some, like the cheese, were slightly processed)—so Kim ordered one. When it came out to her from the kitchen, Kim was starving and sunk her teeth into the Southwestern goodness. But by the third or fourth bite, Kim began to look a little suspicious. She opened the quesa-dilla and asked her friend what sauce was on the appetizer. He told her he thought it was pesto and, at that, Kim darted off to the restroom and *removed* the food from her system as best she could.

Kim is one of nearly twelve million Americans who suffer from an overactive immune system when she ingests a certain food; in other words, she has a food allergy. In Kim's case, she is allergic to pine nuts, which are a key ingredient in pesto and which made that tasty quesadilla a physiological threat. When Kim takes in this allergen, bad things happen to say the least; her tongue and throat start to swell, she has difficulty breathing, and eventually begins to have abdominal cramps and diarrhea.

Kim's pine nut allergy, which is part of the larger tree nut allergy, is one of "the Big Eight" food allergies that account for roughly 90 percent of all food allergies in the United States. The other allergies that comprise the Big Eight are dairy, egg, peanut, seafood, shellfish, soy, and wheat. Some food allergies cause the condition anaphylaxis in sufferers, which leads to 50,000 emergency room visits and some 150-200 deaths each year. The Food Allergy & Anaphylaxis Network describes anaphylaxis as:

An anaphylactic reaction may begin with a tingling sensation, itching, or a metallic taste in the mouth. Other symptoms can include hives, a sensation of warmth, wheezing or other difficulty breathing, coughing, swelling of the mouth and throat area, vomiting, diarrhea, cramping, a drop in blood pressure, and loss of consciousness. These symptoms may begin within several minutes to two hours after exposure to the allergen, but life-threatening reactions may get worse over a period of several hours.

Recovery from anaphylaxis can vary:

> In some reactions, the symptoms go away, only to return
> two to three hours later. This is called a "biphasic reaction."
> Often these second-phase symptoms occur in the respiratory
> tract and may be more severe than the first-phase symptoms.
> Studies suggest that biphasic reactions occur in about 20
> percent of anaphylactic reactions.

It is important to note here that food allergies and intolerances are quite different. Not everyone is allergic to the Big Eight allergens—pine nuts made Kim's body revolt against the quesadilla, but her friend couldn't get enough. As noted in the Introduction, food allergies are distinct from intolerances or toxicities in that allergies are dramatically more dangerous, but more people tend to have intolerances to those foods and if a certain food is toxic, it is toxic to everyone, not just to allergy sufferers. What is striking is that the same foods that cause allergies in 12 million Americans are the same foods that many more are intolerant to and which are toxic generally (in all, nearly one out of every five Americans suffers from some adverse reaction to food and all suffer toxicity from some foods). And they are the same foods that Natural Man avoided because it lessened his chance of survival. Could food allergies be that nature is trying to tell us something? Perhaps we shouldn't eat those foods?

That may just be the reaction you get after reading the following descriptions. We will take a look at the Big Eight food allergens and see the history of each as something edible and what damage it can do with regard to toxicity, intolerance, and allergies. Below is a list of each of the Big Eight (in alphabetical order) along with pertinent recommendations for dietetic intake. If you feel you might be allergic to any particular food, please read the section for diagnosis in the appendix. It may be vital that you stop consuming the food immediately.

If you think you may be intolerant to a particular food, you may want to consider an elimination diet of the food item completely from your diet. An elimination diet basically consists of (1) checking for symptoms of inconsistent energy, appetite, bowel function, mood, sleep, skin (rash, breaking out), indigestion, or anything suspicious and record your findings every day during a week-long diet excluding the food and two days following. (2) If you notice a substantial decrease in symptoms, extend the elimination for one year to control for environmental factors. (3) After one year, you can try to re-introduce the suspect food into your diet. If your symptoms reappear, you can consider yours to be a significant intolerance and should eliminate the food from your diet altogether. A detailed description of the elimination diet can be found in the appendix.

Dairy

Humans, like other mammals, rely solely on mother's milk for sustenance in the first year or so after birth. In order to digest the sugar in milk (lactose), we naturally produce an enzyme called lactase. However, after humans are able to derive nutrition from other sources (solid foods like fruits, vegetables, and that yummy woolly mammoth meat), we naturally lose the ability to produce lactase and, consequently, the ability to digest milk. Our Paleolithic friend Nat had no need for lactase, however, because he didn't drink milk or eat milk products after his first year. He could get all of his nutrition from plants or meat without clinging on to dairy.

But after certain cultures started domesticating animals, they envisioned getting all that they could out of the animals and that included the milk those animals produce. In fact, over a lifetime, a cow's milk represents a substantial amount, if not a majority of the calories derived from the animal. But the problem of lactose intolerance continued to rear its ugly head—it doesn't make much sense to ingest an animal byproduct for nutrition if it makes one sick.

So, Paleolithic chefs extraordinaire kept the milk out in the open until it soured or fermented and subsequently became curdled. As Reay Tannahill described in *Food in History*, "Milk being highly perishable...a few hours would be enough to start it fermenting in the climate of the Near East. Depending upon the temperature and the kind of bacteria in the air, the curds might develop into something pleasant and refreshing, or something quite uneatable even by Neolithic peoples...Throughout much of history, and especially in hot climates, milk has always been most used in one or other of its soured or fermented forms." This fermented milk became yogurt in the Balkans, *taetta* (a runny viscous milk which vegetable juices are added to prevent coagulation) in Scandinavia, and *dahi* (a milk yogurt with live culture) in India.

Fermentation and souring lets people digest milk products after they've stopped producing a substantial amount of lactase, but one problem remains: since milk is new on mankind's diet, we haven't evolved to handle all of what we take in with dairy products. Most notable are the numerous hormones and harmful macronutrients present in milk products.

Regarding the hormones, insulin-like growth factors

(IGFs) are thought to cause cancer and studies have shown that increased intake of milk products increases IGFs (specifically IGF-1) in adults. Researchers say that further study needs to be done to prove the connection between milk and cancer, but there are certainly troubling initial findings, though some groups (notably the Citizens for the Integrity of Science) have rejected all claims of the link between milk and cancer.

Besides the high amount of animal hormones present in milk products, they also contain high amounts of fat and cholesterol, macronutrients vital for the health of infants and newborns, but detrimental to adults. Over time, fat contributes to obesity and cholesterol contributes to coronary artery disease and other cardiovascular problems. One cup of whole milk mozzarella cheese (shredded) contains 30 percent of the Recommended Daily Allowance (RDA of a 2,000 calorie diet) of cholesterol and 74 percent of the RDA for saturated fat.

Along with the everyday issues presented with dairy consumption, one segment of the population suffers from milk allergy (different from lactose intolerance). The principal symptoms of milk allergy are gastrointestinal, dermatological and respiratory. These can translate to: skin rash, hives, vomiting, diarrhea, constipation and distress. The clinical spectrum extends to diverse disorders: anaphylactic reactions, atopic dermatitis, wheeze, infantile colic, gastroesophageal reflux (GER), oesophagitis, allergic colitis and constipation. The symptoms may occur within a few minutes after exposure in immediate reactions, or after hours (and in some cases after several days) in delayed reactions. As usual, if you think you may have an allergy to milk, stop consuming it and consult a physician.

Evo-Diet Recommendation

With so many problems associated with dairy consumption, it's hard to believe it's as popular as it is. Its popularity may stem from its high calorie and nutritional content and because dairy products just taste so good. But alas, the negative aspects of dairy products may finally be catching up to us as a population. While further study of the link between milk products and cancer continue, it would be wise to limit intake of the category.

Some cultures already do without. The Chinese, for instance, abhor milk and milk products are noticeably missing from all traditional Chinese plates (the average consumption per capita per year is under 5 kg for urban Chinese and 0.6 kg for rural Chinese). Anthropologist Marvin Harris attributes this to the fact that throughout history, the Chinese never domesticated cattle and thus never took to the dairy byproduct. Whatever the reason, the Chinese don't consume milk products and they could be much healthier for it. The life expectancy at birth for a Chinese person is 71.4 years while the expectancy for a milk-loving Indian neighbor is nearly 10 years less at 62.5 years.

If you're not allergic to dairy, you can probably handle a small amount of milk products in your diet without ill effect, but mass quantities could lead to severe problems. Take low-fat or skim milk product options when available and limit the overall amount of intake to one or two servings a day to limit the side effects. Of course, you can simply eliminate dairy from your diet altogether much in the same way that the Chinese or vegans do (vegans eliminate all animal products from their diet). It's not an easy task to avoid milk, cheese, most breads, butter, and, most important of all, ice cream, but it is possible.

And if you're concerned about malnutrition from avoiding dairy, don't be; many vegetables contain high levels of the nutrients that milk provides like calcium (see spinach).

Egg

Eggs are a great source of protein and nutrients and easily obtainable as the animals that produce them are neither dangerous nor particularly smart. Eggs have been a culinary treat throughout human history so it's not clear when egg consumption began, but we do know something about it. Raw eggs have a high chance of containing the enterobacteria salmonella, which causes abdominal discomfort, diarrhea, and sometimes even typhoid fever. The infection isn't usually deadly but affects an estimated 1.4 million cases annually.

A surefire way to avoid salmonella is to cook the egg or the recipe including egg. 10 minutes at 75°C (167 °F) at the center is enough to kill off most of the bacteria that might occur in the food. Prehistoric man probably attempted to eat the nutritious egg raw, but perhaps suffered for it with high incidences of salmonella. After all, if there are 1.4 million cases of the food poisoning a year now when most people make sure to cook their eggs, imagine the high incidences of the condition before cooking. It is likely, then, that Natural Man did not consume eggs or else he risked dehydrating himself and becoming deathly ill from salmonella poisoning.

Once cooking became common practice, however, eggs as a culinary staple did catch on. As Maguelonne Toussaint-Samat explains in her *History of Food*:

Farming the prolific chicken has allowed us to make eggs
a part of our diet without harming its reproductive cycle.
However, the very few ancient Greek recipes to mention
eggs date from after the time of Pericles, when the chicken
was introduced to Africa. It took some times for the habit of
using eggs in cooking to catch on. We do hear of thagomata,
made from egg whites, and various stuffings using egg yolks.
On the other hand the classic cake offered as a sacrifice
by the Romans, the libum, called for one egg to a pound of
flour. In the Roman period pastry cooks made much use of
eggs for desserts as well as cakes. Apicius (25 BC) invented
baked custard: milk, honey and eggs beaten and cooked in
an earthenware dish on gentle heat. Eggs really made their
way into the kitchen with Apicius, who mentioned them
frequently in the Ars Magirica. Beaten eggs were used as a
thickening and to bind sauces and ragouts; hardboiled eggs
became an ingredient of various dishes, sometimes with
cheese, but here is no evidence that eggs were eaten just as
they were, as a dish in themselves. This does not mean that
they were not so eaten; it could simply indicate that they
were not thought interesting enough for special mention.

But evolution constantly rears its ugly head and has
prevented us from enjoying eggs as much as we would have
liked. Since Nat didn't evolve eating eggs, our bodies aren't
completely ready for them. The high amounts of cholesterol in
eggs can lead to health problems such as atherosclerosis and
coronary artery disease (CAD), both of which increase the risk
of heart attack. More immediate for some people, eggs cause
allergic reactions.

There are antigens in both egg whites and the yolk,

which affect different populations and people who are allergic to the antigens in egg whites may be able to consume the yolk and vice versa. Egg allergies occur mostly in children, most of who outgrow the allergy by the age of five. Some people remain affected by the allergy throughout their life.

Evo-Diet Recommendation

If you do not have an allergy to eggs, they can be a rich source of nutritious protein and vitamins. The down side is the extra cholesterol baggage that accompanies eggs. You can avoid the high cholesterol price of an ovo-diet by simply using the egg whites, which contain no cholesterol but still contain a good amount of protein, riboflavin, selenium, and potassium, instead of the entire egg. By doing this, however, you eliminate the nutritious yolk, which is chalk full of vitamins and minerals. The optimum combination for any recipe would be to include one complete egg (with whites and yolk) and the rest just egg whites.

Peanut

When Europeans landed in the New World five hundred years ago and discovered the peanut plant, they didn't know what to think. Explorer Bertolomé de las Casas equated the species to filbert nuts (hazelnuts) without the shell but also noticed similarities between the odd plant and beans, sweet peas, and chick peas. Contrary to its name, the peanut is not a nut; it is a legume but it has a strange characteristic. Unlike other legumes, the peanut's ovary is fertilized above ground, and then the stem pushes the flower underground where the peanut grows into the edible item we're familiar with.

Soon after its discovery, the Europeans found that the peanut was rich in fat and fiber as well as a number of micronutrients. Peanut oil was also extolled as quite good. With the aid of Spanish explorers, the plant soon spread from the Americas to Asia and Africa and became a wildly popular food despite some culinary snobs thumbing their noses to the peanut's "mediocre taste." Now the groundnut, as it's also called, is one of the world's most popular crops, growing in 100 countries and on all habitable continents. Some pundits have even gone as far as to claim that the peanut saved Europe and other populations from a disastrous shortage of food around the time of its discovery.

In a way, the easy-to-grow and highly caloric peanut did help feed the world and perhaps even extend the lives of otherwise hungry humans. But in another way, the strange plant food has limited life for many. The most recognized incidences of the damaging properties of the peanut come from new headlines, which indict peanuts or peanut butter in the tragic deaths of allergy sufferers or salmonella victims. Indeed, peanuts can cause allergic reactions like vomiting, heart palpitations, cardiac arrest, and sometimes even death. And it doesn't take much to ignite an allergic reaction; in 2005, a Canadian girl who was allergic to peanuts died after kissing her boyfriend who had eaten peanuts.

However, you don't have to be allergic to peanuts or eat peanut butter contaminated with salmonella (which can attack any number of other foods), for them to be a threat. Peanuts contain high concentrations of toxic (or, less alarmist-sounding, non-nutritive) lectins. Lectins are proteins that bind together with other proteins or sugars and lead to clumping of cells in the intestines and elsewhere in the body. Lectins are present in pretty much all foods, but some plants have more than others, and more lectins means greater chance of inflammation and toxicity.

As A. Pusztai summarized in his book *Plant Lectins*, the common toxic effects of lectins (including those found in peanuts) are:

1. High degree of resistance to gut proteolysis.
2. Binding to brush border cells; damage to microvillus membrane; shedding of cells; reduction in the absorptive capacity of the small intestine.
3. Increased endocytosis; induction of hyperplastic growth of the small intestine; increased turnover of epithelial cells.
4. Interference with the immune system; hypersensitivity reactions.
5. Interference with the microbial ecology of the gut; selective overgrowth.
6. Direct and indirect effects (hormones, etc.) on systemic metabolism.

In other words, lectins are hard to break down, so they persist and bind to the intestine walls, damage the lining and pass through the gut wall into general circulation. Lectins have been associated with colitis, Crohn's Disease, Celiac-Sprue (more on this in the section on wheat), Irritable Bowel Syndrome (IBS) and gut permeability.

All of this is no surprise. Foods that are high in lectin content have only recently been introduced to humankind's diet. Peanuts weren't widely eaten until their discovery in the

16th century—a relative blink of the eye on an evolutionary scale—and humans simply have not evolved to digest the lectins that they contain.

Evo-Diet Recommendation

While peanuts have much in the way of nutrients, they also contain the non-nutritive lectins that harm us in innumerable ways. Most people can handle a small does of these toxins; after all, most foods contain some lectins. But a few edible plants and animal byproducts contain considerably high amounts and the peanut is one of those. Moreover, some may experience symptoms of lectin intolerance like the aforementioned Celiac-Spruce disease or IBS. Some people are allergic to peanuts (different from intolerant) and are at risk of serious immediate side effects by consuming peanuts.

Again, if you think you may have an allergy to peanuts, it is vital that you stop consuming anything with peanuts in them (manufacturers of processed foods are labeling their products with allergy content including peanuts) and seek out a medical evaluation. Otherwise, peanut and lectin intolerance can be self-diagnosed.

It has been shown that soaking, sprouting, cooking, and fermenting peanuts inactivates much of the lectin content, but not all. So, if you're going to eat peanuts, we recommend that you avoid eating them raw and if you experience digestive problems after eating heated peanuts, we recommend an elimination diet of seven days without peanuts or peanut products (cooked or uncooked).

It's important to note that peanuts and the soybean (detailed below) are in the same family and have much of the same allergic properties. It is recommended that you avoid both foods in your elimination diet to ensure validity.

Seafood

I can't imagine having to forgo baked salmon, seared ahi, or pecan crusted tilapia my entire life, so the seafood allergy sufferers elicit the most sympathy from me. Fish as a food is one of the healthiest and tastiest items on the menu and it's been in our collective human diet since the dawn of man (there is even evidence of humans eating fish 380,000 years ago), but there are those unfortunate ones who are allergic to seafood. In fact, the Food Allergy and Anaphylaxis Network (FAAN) has published studies showing some 6.6 million Americans are affected by seafood allergies. They are mostly adults (3 percent compared with 1 percent of children), and the reaction can be very serious: hives, wheezing, throat tightness, or anaphylactic shock.

Evo-Diet Recommendation

Unlike most other food allergens, seafood has been eaten since humans first had hunger pangs, so it can be seen as a food we've evolved to eat. If you don't have an allergy to seafood, we strongly recommend incorporating some fresh fish into your diet.

Shellfish

Shellfish allergies have much in common with seafood (fish) allergies, but are considered separately because one can be al-

lergic to one and not the other. It probably took culinary cavemen a bit longer to start eating shellfish (e.g. lobster, oysters,
mollusks, crab), but they have been in our diet long enough to
have evolved to eating them. As Katherine Szabo described in
her *Prehistoric Shellfish Gathering*:

> At present, the earliest evidence for shellfish consumption
> comes from a 300,000-year-old site in France called Terra
> Amata. This is a 'hominid site' as modern Homo sapiens did
> not appear until around 50,000 years ago. Other early sites
> include caves and open sites from South Africa dating from
> 130,000 to 30,000 years ago, the Cantabrian coast of Spain
> (50,000 to 40,000 years ago), Vietnam (33,000 to 11,000
> years ago), Australia (35,000 years ago) and the Bismarck
> Archipelago in Papua New Guinea (35,000 years ago).

Clearly, we humans have enjoyed shelled sea life for quite
some time and reaped in the rich nutrients of the food. Thus,
it's an anomaly that people should be allergic to them, but that
is the case and the condition usually results in hives, major
redness and swelling below the skin (angioedema), or anaphylactic shock. Recent studies have shown that 2 percent of adults
have shellfish allergy.

Evo-Diet Recommendation

Like seafood, shellfish is very healthy and humans have generally evolved to eat them. If you do not have a shellfish allergy,
there is very little reason for concern about including shellfish
in your diet. Lobster and shrimp, among other shellfish, are
nutritious high-protein foods perfect for the post-hunt meal for

you modern hunter/gatherers. Shellfish tends to be high in cholesterol, but can be integrated healthily into a diet once or twice
a week.

Soy

It's unclear exactly when humans began cultivating the soybean, but many scholars attribute the feat to North China during the Shang Dynasty (1700 B.C. – 1100 B.C.). By the first
century A.D., soy cultivation had spread to South and Central
China and was quickly becoming a staple crop. Like peanuts,
soybean cultivation exploded worldwide with the help of the
explorers from Spain, Portugal, and Britain during the Age of
Discovery, first to Japan, Indonesia, and Southeast Asia, then to
Europe and the Americas.

The main derivations from soybeans were miso soup,
soy sauce, and, of course, tofu. By 1665, European explorers
were fascinated with the use of soy as Friar Domingo Navarre-
te, a Jesuit traveling in China at the time, described it, "They
drew the milk out of the Kidney-Beans and turning it, make
great Cakes of it like Cheeses . . . All the Mass is as white as
the very Snow . . . Alone it is insipid, but very good dress'd as
I say and excellent fry'd in Butter."

Soy products are tasty, full of protein, and inexpensive
and those qualities helped feed billions of people in Asia and
elsewhere in the last thousand years or so. However, like other
foods in this list, humans did not evolve to digest soy fully and
the bean contains many substances named anti-nutrients by the
soy industry. These anti-nutrients include protease inhibitors,
phytic acid, soy lectins (or hemagglutinins), and soyatoxin.
When soy is processed, it also accumulates nitrosamines. Here
are brief descriptions of each:

Protese inhibitors: substances that can interfere and retard the natural breakdown of protein in the digestive tract. Researchers have shown that protese inhibitors may cause cancer in test animals, but others claim that, in humans, protese inhibitors actually reduce the incidence of colon, prostate, and breast cancer in humans.

Phytic acid: chemical that binds to minerals in one's digestive tract and keeps the body from absorbing those minerals (especially zinc, calcium, and magnesium).

Soy lectins: like the lectins in peanuts, soy lectins (hemagglutinins) are substances that clump together red blood cells in humans and in other animal species, and significantly suppress growth.

Soyatoxin: a substance that is immunologically related to canatoxin, which induces convulsions and death in lab animals when injected, but is inactive if given orally. This indicates that the toxin is deadly if enough get into the bloodstream, but digestion prevents a sufficient amount to get through the gut lining.

Nitrosamines: during processing, soy products generate nitrosamines, which, studies have shown, may play a role in the development of nasopharyngeal carcinoma and other cancers.

On top of toxins like these, soy products also cause serious allergic reactions in a large portion of the population. While soy allergy sufferers number far fewer than those with other food allergies, studies show that up to 600,000 Americans may be affected.

It's clear from the description of the soy toxins that there are serious repercussions from a diet heavy in soy products. So, why is it that populations who eat so much of it (Chinese and Japanese for instance) are so healthy on average and live longer than their Western counterparts who don't nearly eat as much soy products? The answer is a familiar one with regard to food allergens: fermentation. The popular foods derived from soy (miso, soy sauce, tofu, tempeh (fermented soy cake), natto, and fermented soy milk) all go through a process of heating, which eliminates much of the toxic content of the bean and leaves a lot of the nutritious goodness.

Evo-Diet Recommendation

There is a lot of contradictory information in the zeitgeist about soy products. Soy is toxic; soy is a tonic. Tofu will save the world; soy will lead to cancer. The main reason for this is that soy products cover a vast array of foods, from edemame and soy sauce at the sushi restaurant to fractionated soybean protein and soynut butter from your local food manufacturer. While traditionally processed soy products are well fermented to remove toxins, the mass-produced soy products that use denatured soy protein usually do not. The rule of thumb here is to avoid soy products that start with a capital letter (i.e. a commercial brand) and products that have TVP, TSP, soy isolate, or denatured soy protein in them and stick with traditional soy foods like miso and tofu).

Tree nut

The almond is native to the area in southern Asia that stretches from India to the Mediterranean and since the Bronze Age of about 4000 B.C., its popularity has spread throughout the world. Almonds can be crushed to produce extract, ground up to produce flour, or eaten raw and this versatility has pushed demand to nearly 2 million tons annually and is why the almond is California's sixth largest cash crop. But the almond as one of the world's favorite foods almost didn't happen.

Almond trees come in two distinct types, one often with white flowers that produces a sweet nut, and one with pink flowers that produces a bitter nut. Farmers chose the former to contribute to many culinary masterpieces, but the latter—the bitter almond—contains about four to nine milligrams of the deadly poison cyanide per almond. Cyanide is a colorless but extremely poisonous and highly volatile chemical that would turn a prehistoric caveman into a suffocating, burning mess if consumed. Needless to say, not too many cavemen or women took the chance in eating almonds because of the risk of melting innards. But after cultivation began in early Neolithic times, daring chefs of the day ventured into the realm of the tree nut to find edible versions of the almond and happened upon the sweet version, which they eventually grew and proliferated throughout the civilized world.

But, as this brief history shows, we humans didn't evolve to eat the almond; we evolved the almond in order to eat it (in a process called cultural selection). The same applies to most of the plants in the entire tree nut family, which, besides almonds, includes Brazil nuts, cashews, hazelnuts, macadamia, pecans, pine nuts, pistachios, and walnuts. Raw cashews and Brazil nuts are protected by urushiol (the poison in poison ivy) on their shells, and walnuts are toxic to horses and dogs (not humans however). If you saw your Stone Age friends trying to eat the nut off a tree and ending up with an itchy swollen esophagus or a dead dog, you would probably start looking for another food source too.

Since we didn't evolve to eat these nuts, it's no wonder that a large portion of the population, like Kim from the beginning of this chapter, is allergic to one or all tree nuts. While most tree nut allergies affect children (6 percent of young children suffer from tree nut allergies whereas 3.7 percent of adults do), many adults suffer as well and must avoid the food throughout their lives. Tree nut allergies account for 13 percent of all food allergies in adults.

Evo-Diet Recommendation

Tree nuts are very healthy as long as the consumer isn't allergic. In general, they don't contain the high amounts of lectins or other non-nutritive substances that other food families have. Conversely, tree nuts are generally rich in vitamins and minerals, high in fiber, and low in sugar. And while the nuts are generally high in fat by content (about half of an almond is fat by weight), the fat is mainly of the monounsaturated kind (the "good" fat). Thus, if you are tree nut allergy free, they can be a great addition to your diet of fresh fruits and vegetables and lean meats.

Wheat

"Wheat," as Tamara Andrews explained in her *Nectar and Ambrosia*, "is the grain that has served as a symbol of ancient harvest deities from the Hittite civilization to the civilizations of ancient Egypt and classical Greece and Rome...Because wheat was the staff of life, people considered it a divine gift, and they made it the focus of ritual from early times." Basically, for much of the ancient world, wheat equaled agriculture in the popular mindset—it was the quintessential plant that was grown and consumed only after domestication. This being said, wheat has been on mankind's menu for quite some time, up to 10,000 years.

As described in the introduction of this part, wheat greatly increased the ability of humans to intake calories. Foods made from wheat were energy-dense, easy to produce and store, and tasty. Wheat allowed the same amount of land in the Fertile Crescent or other areas to reap thousands of times more food than if the plant was left to the ruminants. Instead of relying on seasonal and sparse fruits, vegetables, or tubers, the Neolithic farmers could harvest grain from wheat fields constantly and at a high concentration from their farms.

But wheat was around before 10,000 years ago; why did cultures in the Near East finally start planting wheat when they did? The answer is that wheat was inedible until the practice of cooking became commonplace. Grains in their raw form are highly toxic to humans, but cooking them rendered them edible. And when those imaginative and hungry ancients decided to mix water with the cracked kernels of wild grasses, creating a crude paste, then dropped it on a hot stone until solid, they created the first bread and the rest was history.

Cooking cereals got rid of most of the toxic properties, but as with most of the items in this list, cooking doesn't eliminate all of the issues concerned with consuming the foodstuff. Even after cooking, wheat has substantial amounts of lectins (described in the section on peanuts), gluten (which causes intolerance in around 15 percent of the population), phytates (which inhibit iron absorption), and a number of proteins that cause allergic reactions.

As mentioned above with peanuts, lectins, which bind molecules together in the digestive tract and in the blood stream, can cause damage long term and short term, but are mostly eliminated through cooking. That's not the case for gluten, which persists even after high temperatures are applied to the wheat food. The 15 percent of the population who are gluten intolerant (many cases are undiagnosed) cannot eat wheat (or other grains such as rye and barley) products even after they've been cooked. This condition, also called celiac or coeliac disease, causes gastro-intestinal issues like stomach bloating and cramping, diarrhea, flatulence, constipation etc, neurological symptoms like headache, memory loss, behavioral difficulties, depression, immune system complications like poor resistance to infection, mouth ulcers, arthritis, skin rashes, eczema, psoriasis, itching flaky skin, and general problems like food cravings, tiredness, chronic fatigue, and an unwell feeling. It seems that, with a list of symptoms like that, avoiding wheat might just be the best thing to happen since sliced bread (sorry—I couldn't resist).

Phytates (or phytic acid) in wheat act in much the same way as they do in soybeans; they bind minerals together to inhibit absorption in the digestive process. There have been studies that show phytic acid prevents digestion of zinc, calcium, magnesium and iron. One study focusing on iron showed that as little as 5-10 milligrams of phytate phosphorus inhibited absorption of 3 milligrams of iron by 50 percent. It was also shown, however, that increased intake of ascorbic acid (vitamin C) or meat would offset the negative effects of phytates.

Still more people (0.5 percent of the population) suffer from wheat allergies, which, like the other food allergies come complete with much more dangerous symptoms and conditions: eczema (atopic dermatitis), hives (urticaria), asthma, "Hay fever" (allergic rhinitis), angioedema (tissue swelling due to fluid leakage from blood vessels), abdominal cramps, nausea, and vomiting.

Evo-Diet Recommendation

Wheat is everywhere and it is difficult to avoid especially if you eat man-made foods. But if you have a wheat allergy or are among those suffering from gluten or wheat intolerance, you would greatly benefit from an elimination diet as described in the peanut section. If you don't suffer from wheat allergy or intolerance, it is still recommended that you avoid wheat, barley, and rye products in mass quantities. If you desire to incorporate some grains into your diet, we recommend that they be whole-grain (not refined) and fully cooked as in the case of bread or cereals. Still, with the deleterious effects of wheat, consuming it in any substantial amount will work against your overall nutrition. A slice of whole wheat bread is better than a serving of French fries with mayonnaise, but you may want to stick with something that we were designed to eat (like carrots or broccoli) instead of either.

Adverse reactions can be devastating to sufferers and can turn something that's supposed to be life giving into something that makes life unbearable, both physically and emotionally. As Dr. Paul Enck wrote in a study published in the World Journal of Gastroenterology, "Adults and children suffering from food allergy show impaired quality of life and a higher level of stress and anxiety." Those aware of food allergies or intolerances already know the trouble that they come with, but many don't realize that certain foods could be causing a lower standard of living. By familiarizing one's self with the history and nature of food allergens, you will be more attuned to your diet and closer to eating how you were designed to eat.

Part Six

The Evolution Diet

(It's Time To Evolve)

"They are sick that surfeit with too much, as they that starve with nothing."

- William Shakespeare

"The only time to eat diet food is while you're waiting for the steak to cook."

-Julia Child

The guy seemed genuinely offended and looked around to see if anyone else witnessed the social atrocity he did, then walked on — miffed. He had a right to be mad because the caveman in the Geico commercial had just seen an insulting ad claiming the advertiser's website was so easy even a *caveman* could do it. I know, the commercials are inane and silly, but I think they're hilarious and the concept is classic — how a caveman would act in today's society. In a sense, The All-Natural and Allergy Free Evolution Diet is promoting a similar concept — how a caveman (or cavewoman) would *eat* in today's society. The analogy has added significance when you take into account the pilot episode of the television series about the characters in the Geico commercials. In it, the three lead cavemen argue about the merits of culturally driven foods like frozen juice bars and fancy coffees while they're in line at a trendy shop serving frozen yogurt with real fruit.

Aside from the latest "fro yo" craze, though, what and how would a caveman eat if he were introduced to our modern culture? Considering he would want to keep to basically the same components of his usual hunter/gatherer diet, what foods from our modern menu would he select and how would he eat them? The answers to these questions are fairly simple, but not obvious, and fortunately, there's actually a little room for that trendy frozen yogurt with real fruit.

Although the science behind The Evolution Diet is complex, the basic principles are so easy, even a caveman could follow them (sorry, I had to). First, I will go over the basic fundamentals of the diet, then go into an extensive day-to-day plan for the average person. I will follow that with some supplementary concepts to consider while you are eating to evolve so that you may maximize your potential health.

The thought of a new, life-long diet may seem daunting, but you *can* make the change and the rewards are well worth the effort. If you will yourself for a couple days, eventually you will regain the natural rhythms of your body and you will start to crave the natural method of eating. Soon, you won't be able to eat any other way because you will enjoy the way you feel so much.

The Fundamentals

In Paleolithic times, cavemen had a pretty rough time maintaining their healthy diet—there were droughts, which removed much of their plant food from the menu, and when hunting, cavemen often had to worry about being hunted *themselves*. Today, however, our menu is astoundingly and unnaturally consistent, as I will expound on in Part Eight. Our wealth and standard of living has enabled us to ensure that we get the proper nutrition we need reliably day-to-day and throughout the year. It stands to reason then, that the main factor preventing the majority of people from attaining perfect health in our society isn't the lack of healthy food or an over-worked populace; it is confusing culture that promotes artificial foods as healthy and convolutes the natural diet of our ancestors with institutions like the balanced meal.

Our culture provides unhealthy calorie-saturated foods and very little time for activities that are beneficial to us like exercise. The average person in our culture will, thus, find it difficult to eat right and exercise. The Evolution Diet addresses both of these problems by promoting more natural foods and a rearrangement of how we eat them. Simply altering your eating schedule will give you more energy when you need it and, more often than not, added drive to exercise when your body tells you to. Both of those effects will lead to improved health and an ideal weight.

If you are trying to accomplish anything our trial dieters were like losing weight, getting more energy, sleeping better, getting rid of daytime lulls in energy, becoming more alert, or just becoming healthier, all you need to do is follow four principles. It may sound too good to be true, but as thousands of Evolution Dieters can attest, it works and it's not rocket science. If you aren't sure what you're looking for in your diet, The Evolution Diet provides a free health assessment tool on our website at http://www.evolution-diet.com. Click on the link to find out "What's your HealthScore" and you will be directed through a short survey that will gather the appropriate information to assess the status of your health. The tool will then provide basic results like your Basal Metabolic Rate, your Body Mass Index, and your HealthScore. It will also provide fundamental diet and lifestyle principles geared personally to you.

Once you begin to get back to the way you were designed to eat, it will be easier for you to work even harder for your health. All you need to do is get the ball rolling, so to speak, and you will be rewarded, almost instantly.

The first step is already taken care of: you've acknowledged that you'd like to change some things in your diet; you wouldn't have bought this book otherwise. Next up, the four main principles of The Evolution Diet:

 The Principles of The Evolution Diet

1. Listen to your body - eat only when your stomach is shrinking, not when a TV commercial tells you to.

2. Appropriate your diet - snack on low-sugar, high-fiber foods throughout the day and fill yourself with a high-protein meal after exercise.

3. Eat from nature and avoid Artificially Extreme Foods - choose apples, not fried Twinkies.

4. Exercise and sleep when your body tells you to - don't fight energy boosts or lulls.

These principles are the key to living a perfectly healthy life and need a thorough explanation. First we will visit principles one through three, then, in a later section, I will address the fourth principle about exercise and sleep.

Listen to Your Body

One of the main causes of poor health, as noted in the previous sections is that people listen to culture instead of their own bodies. They usually find themselves eating a bag of potato chips out of boredom or because culture has made it 'normal', when they should be eating ONLY when they are hungry. Listening to your body instead of society is one of the most important things someone can do to get back to the way they were designed to eat. If people followed this principle alone, they would lose a good amount of unwanted weight and/or feel dramatically better.

The extraordinary thing about this principle is that you don't need any complicated or expensive gadget to be able to follow it and track when it's time to eat; you have an automatic meal timer and calorie counter built in your body. Hunger pangs, the sensation of your contracting stomach or intestines, are your cue to start looking for more food. The trick is to decipher between actual physical hunger pangs and other things that compel us to eat like boredom, stress, or habits such as the mechanical reaction to the lunch bell. This seems obvious, but few people in our Outlook-calendar-dictated-lives actually do it. The key is to eat only when your body is telling you, not for psychological or cultural reasons.

The first principle of The Evolution Diet gets to the heart of the difference between two common words associated with eating: hunger and appetite. Hunger is the physical sensation of discomfort or weakness that is caused by the lack of food, whereas appetite is simply the desire for food. Hunger is the *physiological* need for food and appetite is the *psychological* need for food. The difference is that hunger addresses a real need, whereas appetite addresses an artificial need to eat. To attain the ideal diet, we must eat only when we're hungry, not when we have an appetite for food.

To do this, we must listen to our bodies—physical hunger pangs are the direct indication that your stomach is shrinking as a normal step in digestion and they are your body's way of telling you that it's time to eat. When your stomach does this, your metabolism begins to slow down, which means you begin to lose energy, store fat, and your endocrine system starts to kick in causing unneeded stress. To avoid slowing your metabolism you must satisfy your hunger with a small amount of natural low-sugar, high-fiber food.

That means that people who naturally like to eat constantly are in luck. The Evolution Diet promotes constant snacking throughout the day on natural foods. You can do this because you will not be eating large 1,500-calorie meals every four hours; you will be eating small quantities of moderately difficult to digest foods. As I described in Part Four, natural foods like vegetables, nuts, and fruits tend to be much more difficult to digest than typical fast food like doughnuts or French fries. We are designed to pick at food constantly all day, and we should, as long as the food isn't the super-artificial foods that you would find at the end of a drive-thru or dessert aisle in the grocery store.

The types of food that are perfect for this constant eating in small quantities are low in sugar and high in fiber, or what we will call LoS Hi-Fi foods, and other complex carbohydrates with a moderate amount of fat and protein. But, before you bite into that slab of cardboard next to you, read what tasty snack foods are perfect for this period of the day:

For all of the items above, as well as the rest of the foods we clas-

 LoS Hi-Fi (Low-Sugar, High-Fiber) Foods

- Fresh broccoli with fat-free ranch
- Roasted almonds
- Roasted corn chips with salsa
- Fresh romaine lettuce leafs
- Seasoned sweet peas
- Low-fat gluten-free granola
- Corn tortilla
- Peaches
- Blueberries
- Celery with all-natural cashew butter
- Sweet peppers
- Green beans with seasoning
- Grape tomatoes
- Salted cashews
- Cauliflower with light pear dressing
- Caprese salad
- Jicama salad
- Cucumber with fat-free dressing
- Apple slices
- Fresh spinach with fat-free dressing
- Strawberries
- Oatmeal
- Lightly seasoned popcorn
- Snow peas
- Seasoned rice pilaf
- Carrots and broccoli
- White rice with sweet and sour sauce
- Pears
- Sweet peas with seasoning
- Pita with hummus
- Salad greens with low fat dressing

sify as healthy LoS Hi-Fi foods, it is important to note two things: (1) Healthy serving sizes are a lot smaller than the typical serving sizes promoted by modern culture, and (2) Even the healthy serving sizes (those on the label of each food) are too much to be eaten during a crammed lunch break. In Nat's prehistoric lifestyle, he would have trouble downing much more than a bite or two of the above foods, much less gorging himself with them, but in today's fast-food society, it's not uncommon for someone to three or four times a healthy serving of three or four different kinds of food. Nat followed the shrinking of his stomach, not the ticking of the work clock, by snacking on the above foods all day instead of stuffing himself with them within a certain time period. As a result, Nat was healthier than most of us today.

Case Study: Bettie
Age: 36 Goal: Weight loss

Bettie started the Evolution Diet after 10 years and 80 pounds of weight gain. She had three surgeries to help maintain her weight. She confessed to lack of motivation and, "needless to say, I am not happy with myself."

She picked up The Evolution Diet quickly and took immediately to the snacking portion of it. "I really enjoy just munching on something during work, and although I can't just eat any time, I can whenever I get a hunger pain. I love the types of food I eat at my desk: [no candy] snack mix, and cucumber and tomato salad with fat free Italian dressing. The amazing thing is, I'm probably eating more than I ever have, or at least I feel like it, and I've already lost 15 pounds!"

You will notice when you eat just a couple bites, you almost immediately thereafter lose the sense of hunger. If you listen to your body, it will tell you to leave the rest of the snack for later. Eat the above foods in small, regulated portions so that you don't get to the point when you feel stuffed, or even full. For instance, say you eat an orange and a small bowl of oatmeal with berries for breakfast and the first time you're hungry after that is at 10 am. Eat a handful of roasted almonds with seasoning. In about twenty minutes you may feel a little hungry again—have three bites of steamed broccoli with balsamic vinaigrette and continue in this way until you're no longer getting any hunger pangs. If you spread out what would be a large lunch out over several hours, you will benefit by maintaining a more consistent metabolism, and as a result, a more consistent level of energy and less discomfort from hunger or overfed.

While snacking in the manner described above feels like you're eating more, you're probably eating less. Researchers at Penn State University have shown that eating an apple about 15 minutes before lunch reduces the amount of food taken in at the meal. The apple-eaters consumed over 180 fewer calories (130 calories when you factor in the apple) than their counterparts who refrained from what I call the *appletizer*. Brian Wansink, director of Cornell University's Food and Brand Lab in Ithaca, N.Y. said, "This is great evidence that it's not the calories, but it's the effort of eating that tricks us into thinking we're full." When we're in lunch mode, we're not concerned with eating appropriately, we usually just want to finish off the plate in front of us and do so in the allotted 30 minutes. Snacking, on the other hand, refocuses our attention on our body's clues and allows us to eat only what our body is asking for.

Remember, there is a happy medium between the hunger

pangs you feel and the stretched-stomach feeling you have after eating too rapidly. It is important to maintain this happy medium throughout the day if you want to eat how your body is designed to eat. Eating only when you are hungry and not overeating when you do will take some discipline at first, but once you get the hang of it, you will not want to eat any other way.

Appropriate Your Diet

One of the worst things about the average modern diet is the failure to appropriate and eat specific foods when they're needed and only when they're needed. This aspect also tends to be the most beneficial to one's health and the aspect that most other popular diet plans overlook. We were designed to eat certain foods at certain times because those foods provide our bodies with timely benefits. The Evolution Diet breaks down healthy foods into three categories: complex carbohydrate snacks or LoS Hi-Fi foods, high-energy foods, and high-protein foods. LoS Hi-Fi foods, as described above, provide one's body with sustained energy throughout the day; high-energy foods give one's body a boost before, during, and immediately after exercise; and high protein foods rebuild one's body after exercise and prepare you for sleep. Each healthy food category has a specific time to be eaten according to your activity throughout the day, but there are a number of factors in modern culture working against this appropriation. Cultural superfoods (e.g. wheat, rice, and corn), fast food, and, believe it or not, the balanced meal are just a couple of the agents working against a healthy diet—all of these go against what your body is designed to consume.

Someone may even be eating all-natural and healthy foods,

but if he isn't eating them at the appropriate times — according to activity — he is not maximizing his diet. For example, eating too much sugar before sleep would make one restless at night and tired the next day. Also, eating a large protein meal in the morning may make one sleepy an hour later, only to be combated with three or four cups of coffee.

If you are overweight, nervous, tense, easily stressed, or a horrible sleeper, simply appropriating your diet could do wonders. All of those conditions could be due to the body not getting what it needs with regard to energy and nutrients at the right time. Nat, our friendly caveman, ate specific types of food at specific times and as Omberto, an Evolution Dieter, likes to put it, "There is food for work, food for play, and food for the rest of the day." The food for work is the high-protein meal; the food for play is the healthy high-energy foods; and the food for the rest of the day is LoS Hi-Fi snacks. This is the essence of appropriating your diet.

Good foods must be eaten at the right time to truly be good. For example, an orange is a very nutritious food that provides vitamins that help bolster our immune systems and prevent diseases like scurvy. We can easily employ the energy we get from an orange, and the moderate amount of fiber it contains regulates our digestive tracts. So, an orange should be considered a healthy food.

But, if someone ate five oranges in an hour right before attempting to sleep, it would not be healthy because the easily digested sugars in an orange might make the citrus fanatic shoot around like the Tasmanian Devil while the high acidity in the orange may cause an imbalance of pH in the stomach. This wouldn't make for pleasant sleep. Also possible is an overabundance of vitamin C. All vitamins become toxic at certain levels, and while humans can take in and use a super-high amount of vitamin C (RDA of vitamin

C is 60 mg, while the toxicity level is somewhere around 25,000 mg), it is possible to have too much of it. With all this being said, it is easy to see how eating so-called healthy foods does not always contribute to health. There is validity in the maxim, "one *can* have too much of a good thing". Moderation, as well as appropriation, is the key to eating the way we would naturally eat things.

In the same way that eating too much of a healthy food is bad for you, so is eating certain foods at the wrong time. Both dietary flaws give you something your body doesn't know what to do with. Conversely, it is beneficial to eat certain foods at the right time—the essence of appropriating one's diet. You may have heard of good foods to eat before you sleep like a warm glass of milk or cottage cheese. Just as there are good foods to have before sleep, there are good foods that you should eat throughout the day, during exercise, or when you are tired but don't want to be.

 An Evolution Diet Essential

Humans naturally want a bit of food in their stomachs at all times. But you should replace the Snickers bar with highly fibrous foods to keep the process natural.

Complex carbohydrates are perfect throughout the day because they offer a constant flow of energy—enough to allow the body to perform optimally without spiking blood sugar. Healthy sugars are good surrounding exercise to ensure a sustained, high-energy output. They are also handy when you need a little pick-me-up or when you're feeling tired, but can't afford to sleep. When you are not dependent on sugar and not constantly eating sweets (like many of us do), a natural high-sugar food will kick up your energy before you can say, "maltodextrose."

Of course, the most valuable thing we put in our body—water—should be consumed consistently throughout the day. Especially good times to drink it, though, are before meals and before and after sleep. If you are trying to lose weight, water is a great way to trick your body into thinking that it is fuller than it is. When you mix a tall glass of water with your regular high-protein dinner, you tend to eat less since you feel more of a bulge. Water is more important than fooling your stomach it's fuller than it is and I will describe other benefits later.

A high-protein meal is perfect a short while after exercise and before rest and sleep. Since exercise damages your tissue (most notably your muscles), your body asks for the materials to rebuild that tissue after you are done working out. When you eat protein after exercise, there is a specific need for the amino acids you consume and detrimental protein metabolism, which turns protein into energy and ammonia, is avoided. If your body gets too much protein, which is what happens when you eat it at the wrong time, the body breaks it down and stores it as fat or gets rid of it all together, creating additional toxins in the body. If you eat protein after physical exercise, however, it's beneficial in rebuilding the vital tissues throughout the body.

As touched on in Part Four, there are a number of reasons why a large high-protein meal (i.e. the buffalo you just hunted) makes sense in the evening before rest besides the benefits of rebuilding physical tissue. (1) Protein also makes for a good pre-sleep meal because it usually contains the essential amino acid tryptophan, which brings the energy level down and aids sleep. (2) Protein is digested slower than an equivalent amount of complex carbohydrates, making it ideal to eat before extended periods of rest. (3) A large amount of food makes the consumer more tired immediately following the meal because the thermic effect of food (the amount of energy required to digest food) is higher for a larger meal. Blood rushes to the digestion organs when a large amount of food is present, drawing it from other areas, like one's head, making the eater more tired.

With The Evolution Diet, one can eat to their heart's content around dinnertime, as long as one is eating high-protein foods. Around 70 percent of your dinner, in weight, should be protein, preferably eaten before the carbohydrates; a method of determining this is found in Part Ten. Throughout the day, while consuming a consistent amount of LoS Hi-Fi foods, the Evolution Dieter's metabolism is running evenly. We recommend physical exercise in the late afternoon or early evening (after work is perfect), during which the body is physically stressed. Hunger should subside throughout the physical exercise, but when it returns, we recommend a large meal full of healthy high-protein foods like fish, pork,

 High Protein Meals (main course with side dishes)

- Chicken burrito with black beans and a chipotle salsa
- Grilled turkey salad with low-fat dressing
- Crab-stuffed salmon steaks on a bed of spinach
- Thai chicken crêpe with broccoli and almonds
- Filet mignon steak with cheese artichoke side
- Grilled tuna and bean salad
- Southwestern omelet with tomato, avocado, and honey-glazed ham
- Caesar salad with grilled chicken
- Hamburger lettuce wraps with roasted asparagus
- Pulled pork open-faced sandwich with sweet peas
- Braised leg of duck with Thai curry
- Barbequed chicken with green beans
- Seafood quiche with tomato slivers
- Spinach-stuffed meatloaf with grilled zucchini
- Carne asada and salsa burrito bowl (without the wrap)
- Ham and cheese crêpe with steamed broccoli and cauliflower
- Roasted salmon with macadamia cilantro crust and squash
- Cajun flavored crab legs and lobster tail with whipped cauliflower

or chicken. This change in the digestive process is natural and coincides perfectly with your normal sleep cycles. It should be noted that the size of a high protein dinner should be proportional to the amount of exercise done before.

Let's review. To eat what and how you would naturally eat involves snacking on foods that are low in sugar and high in fiber with a little protein throughout the day to sustain a high and level amount of energy. It is acceptable to eat natural high-energy foods before, during, and after exercise. And a couple hours after exercise and a few hours before sleep, you should fill yourself with a 70 percent protein meal and very little sugar (5 percent at most). Your high-protein meal should be big enough to tide you over through sleep, but if you're hungry after dinner, you should have a high-protein dessert like cottage cheese with a few slices of a peach.

Eat From Nature

When you awake in the morning, The Evolution Diet's snacking/exercise/meal/sleep cycle starts over with moderate intake of complex carbohydrates and a little bit of protein. Breakfast is the beginning of the LoS Hi-Fi snack stage described above and should consist of basically the same foods. Some people may need a little extra boost in the morning. If that's the case for you, you may want to include a small natural, high-energy portion as a supplement, not a tall cup of coffee. One of the main principles in The Evolution Diet is to eat from nature and that means avoiding what is known as Artificially Extreme Foods (AEFs), which are exceptionally dense in calories or any other ingredient like coffee is with caffeine. Although caffeine can be found naturally in many foods,

Case Study: Cindy

Age: 25 Goal: Better sleep, Weight loss

It took Cindy an emergency in the family to alert her to health. Although she has always been relatively healthy, she wanted to eat better. "As a result of my father's stroke (he is ok, in a residential rehab program) my mother and I have decided to try to become healthier together. I have joined a gym and she has started going on morning walks with our dog. The problem is eating. We both have weight to lose (she has much more than I do) and want to eat healthier food, but don't really know where to start or what to change.

"I would love to lose some weight (I just graduated from college and gained a lot of weight while enjoying my senior year), maybe 10 pounds or about that, and get healthy. I just started my first real job but it is not causing too much stress in my life, but I am more stressed than I used to be. And I NEVER sleep well anymore without the help of sleeping pills (which I try not to take more than twice a week and only when necessary, I don't want to become addicted)."

After two years on The Evolution Diet, Cindy has kept the weight down (she has lost about 34 lbs. and has maintained her weight since). She's found the high-protein meal in the evening the key to better sleep. "Since I began eating almost all protein at night after my exercising, I've gotten really tired about 3 hours after the meal. I didn't know a change in diet could do so much to my physical state. The sleep has been unbelievable! I wake up and don't feel like I've just been tossing and turning all night. I feel energetic and spunky in the morning. It's fantastic- I don't think I'll ever change the way I eat now."

Congrats Cindy!

coffee is considered one of the Artificially Extreme Foods because it is easy to achieve an excess intake of one of its ingredients with the modern serving portions.

One coffee bean, found in nature has about 2 mg of caffeine and a relatively unpleasant, bitter taste to it. If someone were to eat coffee beans in nature they would probably get bored after about 5, maybe 10, and they would get a nice little kick from caffeine shortly after (though caffeine takes about an hour to take effect). A person sitting down to a tiny cup of espresso, however, is taking in the equivalent of 50 coffee beans! Of course, one serving doesn't quite suffice for those of us who are used to the medium grande triple shot, iced latte con panna with a little lemon twist. Drinks like those and the most fully loaded beverages at your neighborhood Starbucks have an amazing 330 mg of caffeine! Yikes!

Although caffeine has some immediate benefits to health like increased awareness, increased breathing, and appetite suppression, a diet with caffeine as a major staple is extremely unhealthy. In fact, becoming dependent on the drug will not only decrease your tolerance to stress and exercise, it will also cause irregular heart patterns, increased blood pressure, and aggravation of the digestive tract, which may lead to problems such as ulcers. If you're someone who, "can't live without a few cups of coffee a day," that should be your first indication that the dependence on the drug has started. Your body was not designed to handle such a stimulant constantly.

And the effects of this Artificially Extreme Food can be lasting, if not permanent. Extensive MRI testing by Paul Laurienti of Wake Forrest University has shown an interesting trait about brain activity in heavy caffeine drinkers versus non-caffeine users. It showed that the brain activity of a coffee drinker and a non-coffee drink was relatively the same, but only when the coffee drinkers

Caffeine Content of Various Foods

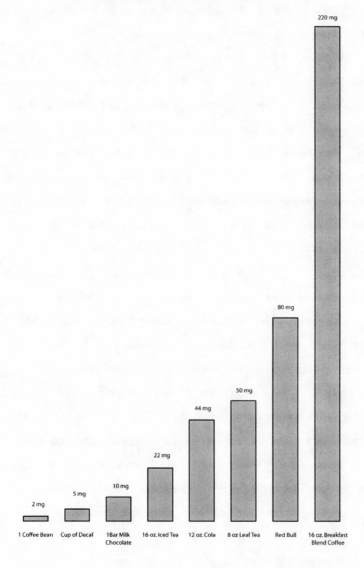

had caffeine in their system. When the coffee drinker didn't have any caffeine or when the non-drinker did, the differences were dramatic. In essence, the body likes a certain level of brain activity and if you are constantly feeding yourself a stimulant, the body will compensate for that and return to the normal level of activity. Laurienti said, "If you regularly get a hefty dose [of caffeine], you need it for your brain to function normally." The psychoactive drug is a nice pick-me-up when you really need it (e.g. when you're driving late at night), but when you become dependent on it, caffeine is actually holding you back.

Coffee is just one in the group of edibles called Artificially Extreme Foods, which I have mentioned a couple times in this book. But despite coffee's extreme nature, there are a number of AEFs that are less healthy and make more sense to avoid, such as fried foods, foods with partially hydrogenated fats, and super-sweet foods like soda pop. The major problem with food like this is that they are more than our body is designed to handle, which is due to the fact that we've made them more condensed or potent than they are in nature. While we can handle just about anything for a short period of time, even AEFs, extended periods of intake of such foods will lead to serious problems like heart disease, high blood pressure, diabetes, or cancer. It is important to avoid these foods whenever possible and eat from nature instead.

Some AEFs have natural origins but are so concentrated or distorted by the time they make it to your plate or cup that they are extremely harmful to our bodies. Oranges are found in nature, but to get an 8-ounce glass of orange juice, one must squeeze 8 to 10 oranges. If someone ate 8 to 10 oranges, he or she would doubt-less be quite full with all the fibrous healthy bits in the rest of the orange. Orange juice is an AEF because it is a source of such high-ly concentrated sugar that it is not natural even though its deriva-tive is natural. The same goes for fried foods. Although saturated fat is found naturally in animals, the concentrated amount that is used to deep fry foods is impossible to find in nature. This leads to a critical point about Artificially Extreme Foods: some, like or-ange juice, can be used as a healthy high-energy food, but others, such as French fries, should be avoided altogether. A good rule of thumb, however, is that the further away from nature a food gets, the worse it is for our bodies.

The Evolution Diet promotes smart ways of taking what you normally eat and rearranging it to optimize your body's mechanical processes, but there are certain foods that you must give up altogether to attain better health. Although there are some instances when you would need to replenish your blood sugar with something like soda pop, this only occurs during extreme physical output (high-level exercising for more than an hour). Even then, it is recommended that you drink something with other benefits than just sugar. Orange and grape juices are high-energy drinks but have other benefits like vitamin C (100 percent of your recommended daily allowance in a small 8 ounce glass). Different drinks can be deceiving also: a can of Coke has nearly twice as many grams of sugar as the same amount of Gatorade, a beverage that

Case Study: Tommy
Age: 25 Goal: Higher Energy

"I'm a healthy guy, for the most part," Tommy explained, "but I can't get rid of these lulls in energy that I get throughout the day. Sometimes it gets so bad, I fall asleep at my desk at the [company]." That's definitely something to be concerned with. When Tommy explained his old diet, it was clear as to why he was experiencing his lulls in energy. He usually had a cup of Bella Vista F.W. Tres Rios® Costa Rica coffee with two sugars from Starbucks in the morning, and maybe a glazed scone if he was feeling hungry. Usually he wasn't, so he was providing a nice little boost of energy for himself—first from the sugar, then from the caffeine. But when that boost was done, he might have been hungry, which would have low-

promotes its energy-boosting effects.

You may be asking, "Well, if I can't eat anything as sweet as a doughnut or as filling as a pound of chili cheese fries, doesn't that take all the fun away from eating?" The answer is NO. When you begin to eat foods the way we were designed, you'll begin to appreciate more subtle flavors in food. In The Evolution Diet you will re-sensitize your taste buds and enjoy a wider range of foods.

I was reminded of the desensitization factor recently on a mountain in Arizona. One day we were heading out to snowboard and ski, and before we hit the slopes, we wanted to get a good amount of energy into us so that we wouldn't get tired throughout the day. I had a bowl of instant oatmeal with a plenty of sugars, a banana, and a couple of glasses of orange/cranberry juice. I then had a bagel that tasted pretty bland, so I put butter and jam on it. I took an additional bagel with me to eat later that day. After a

ered his blood sugar, and he would have no sustainable energy source in his system except for a few grams of complex carbohydrates from the scone. Since he always had his coffee and sugar in the morning, his body had come to depend on that boost. When he became tired a couple hours after, he rightly assessed that the caffeine was wearing off, but he would just drink another cup.

Once he permanently replaced the coffee and scone with a couple slices of buttered toast and an orange, he felt energetic throughout the morning. There were no more lulls caused by the absence of caffeine. He got his energy from the long-term source of complex carbohydrates. This energy source leveled out the spikes and lulls into a constant, healthier supply.

couple runs down the mountain, including about 15 monumental wipeouts, I began to get hungry. I pulled out the bagel and ate a couple bites. To my surprise, the same bagel that had tasted bland a few hours before, tasted extremely sweet on the mountain. Compared to all the sweet foods at breakfast, I hadn't noticed any flavor in the bagel, but a few hours later it tasted almost like candy. The intense sugars we ate in the morning distracted us from tasting the actual flavor in the bagel.

An argument can be made that some Artificially Extreme Foods are appropriate in certain situations, like extreme exercise, except when you're trying to lose excess fat. However, it's important to use common sense; a fried Twinkie, for instance, is not one of those appropriate AEFs, and if you are trying to lose weight, extreme exercise is an opportunity to tap into that excess weight for energy—eating an AEF after extreme exercise will negate some of the positive effects of the workout.

The same principle that applies to sugar with regard to being an AEF goes for fat, as well. We need a moderate level of fat in our diet in order to digest some of the vitamins we eat, but excess fats and, to a lesser extent, excess sugars go directly to storage fat for the next time we're in a famine or something devastating like that. Although real famines are not laughing matters, it can safely be said that most of us in Western culture will not have to go weeks without food, so we don't need that excess fat.

Being able to store fat is a great way for us to live through times without food, but the storage of fat is a very stressful process and it harms us when we take it to the extreme. It is an unfortunate statistic that obese people live an average of 7.1 years less than those with an ideal weight, while just overweight people live slightly longer than obese people. In a shocking report by the University of Illinois at Chicago in 2005, it was reported that life

Case Study: D'Shauwna

Age: 31 Goal: Motivation, Higher Energy

Mrs. White came to The Evolution Diet as a slightly overweight woman who was lacking motivation and didn't really have much energy. "I am not lazy—just have a hard time eating 3 meals a day and my metabolism has stopped, I think. I know that exercise is important to me, but whenever I try to get motivated, I can't imagine anything worse." D'shauwna was used to eating a large mixed-bag of protein and carbohydrates for lunch. After work she expected to feel like exercising. Quite the opposite, D'Shauwna was telling her body that everything was fine in the world of nutrition. In essence, exercise is the component of our modern lives that is linked to the hunting part of hunting and gathering. Since our dieter had filled herself in the middle of the day, that made her feel content without "hunting" for substantial food.

We got D'Shauwna on a routine of eating small amounts of complex carbohydrates throughout the day, and a little sugary boost right before she was going to the gym. Viola, she had, "More energy than [she] ever has had," before exercising. She was shocked, but getting rid of a giant meal in the middle of the day and filling the gaps with small food made her prepared, even excited for exercise.

expectancy for Americans actually decreased for the first time. The main reason for this is the increase in obesity, which afflicts one third of the US population (an additional one third are considered overweight).

The single-most important factor in the overweight epidemic is the abundance of these Artificially Extreme Foods. Studies have shown that the average American diet increased calorie

Some Healthy High-Energy Foods

- Oranges
- V-8 Splash
- Carrots
- Yams with sugar glaze
- Grapes
- Corn Flakes with milk
- Carrot cake
- Strawberries
- All-natural granola bar
- Raisins
- Trail mix with dried fruit
- Peanut butter and Jelly
- Banana pudding with graham crackers
- Orange sorbet
- Bananas

intake by 10 percent from the mid 1970s to the mid 1980s. They didn't see an increase in serving size (however shocking that may seem); they saw an increase in the caloric *density* of foods. When you add that higher caloric density in foods with the enormous sized portions we eat today, it's no wonder that the majority of Americans are overweight.

The bright side of this is that it's never too late for you to correct this problem. You can start with the next bite you eat. The way to do this is eat the way we were designed to eat, not the way the television or our schedules tell us to eat.

Humans naturally want a bit of food in their stomachs at all times. In addition, as we've noted, they can handle large quantities (of protein) when needed. But when you replace the low calorie, high fiber foods found in nature with high density, jam-packed foods like a power bar, there is a problem: you will be hungry in a shorter while than if you had eaten a couple stalks of broccoli, but you will have taken in 10 times the amount of calories. This fact is so simple and obvious, yet is still obscure from the common cognizance.

There are certain dieting techniques out there that focus solely on this aspect of The Evolution Diet. The Pritikin Principle is to eat foods that have lower calorie-per-pound ratios. It is not too hard to see how the further a food is from its natural origins, the more calorically dense and extreme it is. An interesting comparison that demonstrates this principle is the different ways to prepare a staple food for many Americans today: corn. Natural corn off the stalk is a fairly sweet 490 calories per pound, while tortilla chips at the friendly neighborhood Mexican restaurant are 2,450 calories per pound! The difference can be attributed to the addition of fatty oils, but also to the condensed nature of the corn in the chip.

Hunger is an urge telling us to fill up our stomach, and it can be sufficed by something as simple as water. Water is easily digested, however, and a glass of water won't hold back your hunger very long. H_2O, though, is a great supplement to snacks; a couple tasty roasted almonds and a glass of water will make you just as satisfied as if you were to eat a Snickers bar—contrary to the way its advertisers may want to portray the candy, Snickers has easily digested sugars and does not satisfy. Water is also an important supplement when you're eating dried foods like the fruit in a bag of trail mix. Since the fruit is dehydrated it will take you a lot more to fill yourself than if you were eating fresh fruit. Dried foods usually have much higher caloric density than their hydrated counterparts and many dried fruits have added sugar.

One rule of thumb to keep in mind when trying to avoid AEFs is the more processed a food, the less healthy it is for us and the more jam-packed it is with artificially extreme ingredients. After the sample diet in Part Seven, I will further explain the merits of eating from nature.

Part Seven

Sample Diet
(What An Evolved Diet Might Look Like)

"Dieting—it's something most of us do religiously: we eat what we want and pray we don't gain weight."

-Anonymous

For most people looking to begin eating healthier, it helps to see what the actual diet looks like in action. It's one thing to say that it's good to eat LoS Hi-Fi Foods throughout the day and a high-protein meal after exercise and before rest, but what exactly am I supposed eat? Below is a loose guide of what The Evolution Diet: All-Natural and Allergy Free may look like for a typical dieter. This sample diet excludes milk, peanut, soy, and most wheat products to avoid potential toxins. This is by no means meant to be followed strictly. In fact, since the first principle of The Evolution Diet is to listen to your body, guidelines like these—if followed precisely—might very well contradict your natural hunger cycles. That being said, we offer a concise diet history for eight days. Enjoy!

Day 1

Breakfast:
1 orange
1 cup strawberries
Glass of water

Daytime (eaten over a period of 9 hours):
1 cup roasted almonds
Small spinach salad with tomatoes and sunflower seeds with vinaigrette dressing
1 banana
Water

Exercise:
20 minute walk

Dinner:
Salmon steak with teriyaki sauce and a cilantro pesto spread
Whipped cauliflower with seasoning
Water

Day 2

Breakfast:
Small bowl of oatmeal with brown sugar and blueberries
Small glass of orange juice cut with water

Daytime (eaten over a period of 9 hours):
1 cup of grape tomatoes
1 cup of long-grain rice with hot sauce
½ cup of salted cashews

Exercise:
3-mile jog
40 pushups
100 sit-ups

Post-Exercise Snack:
1 can of tuna with lime juice and salt and pepper

Dinner:
10 oz steak fillet with seasoning
Two cups steamed broccoli with cheese
Diet caffeine-free cola
Water
2 "pecan cloud" gluten-free cookies

Day 3

Breakfast:
2 mangos
2 slices of gluten-free French toast with honey
Tall glass of cranberry juice cut with water

Daytime (eaten over a period of 9 hours):
Small cup of yogurt with gluten-free granola
2 cups fresh snow peas and jicama
1 cup chai tea with flavoring
Water

Exercise:
2 hours of housework

Dinner:
Small plate of gluten-free meatloaf
Glass of red wine
Half cup of cottage cheese with peaches for dessert

Day 4

Breakfast:
2 slices of apricot and almond bread (gluten-free)
Small cup of watermelon fruit salad
1 small bowl of gluten-free granola with rice milk

Daytime (eaten over a period of 9 hours):
2 cups mixed vegetables with pear and champagne dressing
1 apple

Exercise:
1 hour of yoga

Post-exercise snack:
1 glass of rice-protein smoothie

Dinner:
Large buffalo chicken wrap (gluten-free wrap) with cheese, lettuce
and tomato
Tomato, cucumber, feta cheese salad with low-calorie Italian dressing
Water

Day 5

Breakfast:
Small bowl of cream of wheat with light cane sugar
Small glass of cranberry juice cut with water

Daytime (eaten over a period of 9 hours):
2 cups mixed nuts
1 cup of fresh cherries
15 sticks celery with all-natural almond butter

Exercise:
20 minute walk

Dinner:
Egg-white omelet with peppers and mushrooms
2 slices of ham
Water

Day 6

Breakfast:
1 cup pineapple
chunks
1 egg muffin
(no flour) with
butter and fresh
preserves

 An Evolution Diet Essential

Listen to your body when deciding to eat.
Just because there are five more berries left
in the carton, that doesn't mean you have to
eat them if you're not hungry.

Daytime (eaten over a period of 9 hours):
1 can green beans with seasoning
10 carrots bites
½ cup of walnuts
Water

Exercise:
40 minute walk

Dinner:
Small mixed greens salad with zero fat Italian dressing
Cajun-flavored Alaskan crab legs
Shrimp cocktail
2 small lobster tails
(treat yourself every once in a while :D)

Day 7

Breakfast:
Bowl of yogurt with fresh blackberries
Small glass of apple juice cut with water

Daytime (eaten over a period of 9 hours):
Small Greek salad
2 cups grape tomatoes
Half bag of light popcorn
1 cup green tea

Exercise:
40 minute walk

Dinner:
Large Caesar salad
2 ham and cheese crêpes (with gluten-free flour) with spicy tomato
sauce

Day 8

Breakfast:
3 celery sticks with hazelnut butter and honey
Small glass of apple juice

Daytime (eaten over a period of 9 hours):
Half bag of light popcorn
2 bananas
Small spinach salad with cheese and oil and vinegar dressing
Water

Exercise:
3-mile jog
40 pushups
100 sit-ups

Post-exercise snack:
1 mango
Small house salad

Dinner:
2 crab cakes
1 large swordfish steak with capers and lemon sauce
Mixed steamed vegetables with seasoning
2 glasses of wine
Small bowl of cottage cheese with peach slices

Part Eight
Live Off the Land
(Become a Modern Hunter/Gatherer)

"Now I see the secret of the making of the best persons. It is to grow in the open air and to eat and sleep with the earth."
- Walt Whitman

"All wild plants are edible—at least once."
-Anonymous

In late August 1870, an expedition into the heart of the previously uncharted Yellowstone region of Wyoming commenced. A city man and somewhat-scholar named Truman Everts made the decision to join the exploring party, which was comprised of 19 men and their 40 horses. Everts was by no means a professional outdoorsman, but he felt at ease on the trek into the wild because of the large contingent that accompanied him — little did he know that venture would nearly cost him his life.

In mid-September, Everts separated from the main group and was forced to camp alone. Confident he would find the others the next morning, the gentleman-turned-woodsman rested assured that night, unaware of the adventure that was to come. The next morning, Everts rose early and headed out with his horse in the direction he had been traveling earlier, but was somehow turned around and never caught up to the main company. At one point, he made a major mistake — he left his horse untied while scouting ahead on rough terrain and the horse bolted. The horse took with it Everts' guns, blankets, and food; and Everts was left to fend for himself in one of the most dangerous and extreme eco systems in the world.

Things started out well as the novice frontiersman used his book knowledge of wilderness to guide him in his survival. Steering clear of the bears, mountain lions, and wolves that proliferated the area and the highly acidic sulfuric liquids that mixed with the freshwater, Everts found nourishment in small animals and a partially edible thistle plant with a spiny skin and a fairly tasty root. He even was able to start a fire with his opera glass by intensifying the rays of the sun on a patch of dry tinder.

Unfortunately, things weren't all peaches and cream for the nineteenth century Everts in this land of geysers and evergreens. The mountain autumn weather began to pound Everts with cool temperatures and thunderstorms. To prevent from getting hypothermia, he sometimes slept near the scalding thermal pools and volcanic mud found in the region; at one point he fell in and seared his skin. He also slept through a forest fire that had apparently been caused by him and ended up burning much of his hair off before he awoke. To make things worse, the thistle plant that he took as his staple food (now called the Everts thistle, in honor of the unwitting naturalist) began to produce unpleasant digestive problems. Malnourished and isolated, Everts began to have hallucinations.

More than a month had passed since his separation and Truman Everts was in a bad state—almost fifty pounds lighter, wounded in numerous places, and seeing things that weren't there. Finally, a two-man search party found the hapless Everts, who they thought was a wounded bear at first, crawling around on the ground. Everts made it through the ordeal and was able to live a long and prosperous life—even siring a child in his eighties.

This amazing story reveals a dramatic fact about the state of modern humans: we're nearly helpless in the wild. Granted, the conditions that Everts faced were extraordinarily harsh, but he probably was more in touch with how to survive off of nature than 99 percent of Western society today. Can you imagine being thrown into a situation like Everts—alone in the wild with nothing to eat but what was around you? It's a scary thought for most of us who wouldn't be able to spot an edible food unless it was in the grocery store with a price tag next to it.

Based on our culture's widespread ignorance of survival skills, it's hard to believe that we all came from hunter/gatherer societies just a couple thousand years ago. If nature is based on survival of the fittest, how did we survive for so long as *un*fit as we are? The answer is, of course, that we were able to manufacture our food through agriculture, and the knowledge of how to find natural plants and how to hunt game has been replaced with knowledge of how to drive a car to the store and how to microwave a dinner. It's not that today's humans are incapable of living off the land; we're just seriously out of practice.

 An Evolution Diet Essential

Prehistoric Man lived for hundreds of thousands of years without help from the FDA. Living off the land like our ancestors can be healthy by increasing the variety of edibles and increasing appreciation for food itself.

While our culture has forced a new unnatural diet on us, we have yet to evolve it. As described in Part Two, we're still designed to eat like hunter/gatherers, and the fact that we eat a modern diet instead is showing up on our waistline and on the waiting list at the doctor's office. All is not lost, however. We can regain the natural eating methods of our ancestors and recover the healthy lives they led. Living off the land, as the robust !Kung from Part One do, is a guaranteed way to eat natural foods and in turn, eat what we were designed to eat.

The first step to recapturing the eating methods of our ancestors or modern hunter/gatherers is to learn about what they ate. American history is chalk full of instances in which North Americans (Indians) taught European settlers or early American tourists how to eat off the land, an education that consequently saved many lives. The Nez Perce of Northern Idaho helped sustain Lewis and Clark on their first expedition across the American continent with dried salmon and a bread made out of a native flower called camas. Early settlers to California were treated to a staple food for the Yosemite Valley residents, delicious acorn mush. And, of course, English settlement of North America would have been delayed a hundred years or so if it weren't for the support of the Narragansett tribe members who provided the Massachusetts Pilgrims with supplies of corn for their first winter on an unfamiliar continent.

Ignorance of nature can be fatal when venturing off into new lands as the aforementioned travelers did—but most of us aren't venturing off into new lands and, if we are, there will probably be a McDonald's and a Starbucks in that new land. Two distinct groups of people, however, are still interested in living off the land despite the lack of necessity in doing so: (1) a wacky breed of pessimists called survivalists and (2) those who simply don't want lose touch with nature. Survivalists are the small populations of cynics that have made strides to prepare for a natural disaster, an international calamity, or otherwise extremely disruptive event. These ultra-prepared individuals are experts on what to do in case something bad happens: how to build a makeshift shelter, how to protect one's self from military aggression, and how to live off the land. Television shows like Discovery Channel's *Man Versus Wild* documents one man's missions to use survival techniques to travel through harsh environs, all the while doing unappealing things like extracting drinking water from elephant dung and scavenging off a zebra carcass.

The other groups of people who are interested in survival techniques are those who want to know how to live off the land strictly on principle. Conn Iggulden and Hal Iggulden, authors of *The Dangerous Book for Boys* explain that hunting for food is good for the modern boy (as well as his father) in order to get in touch with nature. "If you buy a pork chop, we feel that you should realize what has gone into providing that meat for you." They say. "In a sense, killing for food is a link with ancestors going back to the caves." So, in their popular book, they describe how to hunt a rabbit and, incidentally, how to cook the meat and tan the skin of the little fuzzy critter.

The Iggulden brothers are right about the value of hunting—most of us eat meat daily but have no idea what it's like to hunt or kill an animal—and this is an ethical problem that vegetarians bring up time and time again when trying to convince people to forgo their carnivorous ways. If you can't stomach seeing the production of meat, isn't it reasonable that you shouldn't be able to literally stomach that meat? Likewise, if you don't know what it takes to procure plant food from nature, doesn't it stand to reason that your food choices could very well be altogether unnatural? If someone isn't able to spot an edible plant in the wild, how can they be sure that what they take off of the salad bar is appropriate? These questions go to the heart of a major problem in today's culture: we just don't know what we're putting in our bodies.

This uncertainty leads to the consumption of extremely unhealthy ingredients (e.g. partially- hydrogenated oils) and a general ignorance of the effect of our diets have on our. We all should be aware of what the foods we eat are made of and much of that goes back to identifying it in nature and being able to produce it oneself. The Evolution Diet doesn't require you to cook all of your own food from the ingredients you can find on walks through the wilderness, but living off the land is extremely helpful in learning how we were designed to eat. It is also helpful in appreciating the kind of smorgasbord we have splayed out before us every meal and eliminating the waste that so commonly accompanies this indulgence. When I see plates and plates of food thrown away at restaurants, I'm reminded of the film *Cast Away*, in which Tom Hanks' character struggles for months to learn how to procure food for himself after being stranded on an island. When he returns to civilization, he's amazed by the abundance of food (and waste) at a banquet in his honor.

Trying to find food in the wild will make the process of food consumption today look astonishingly easy and probably excessive. Picking blackberries, for instance is a fun activity but it can be arduous and painful too if you end up on the wrong end of a blackberry bush thorn. In an hour of picking, you can gather enough for a day's worth of fruit, but it isn't easy and it's certainly not like going to the store and picking up a little plastic container full of the delicious treats. To truly know what we should be eating, it's worthwhile to look into actually becoming a part-time hunter/gatherer.

Living off the land

Hundreds, perhaps even thousands of hunter/gatherer societies across the globe were and are able to live healthy lives from what they can find in nature. But what exactly were and are they eating? As explained in Part Two, they're mainly eating whatever is around them: berries, vegetables, fruit, small animals, occasionally a tasty six-legged creature, and large game. One way to determine particular foods that hunter/gatherers ate before culture is to examine the staple food for tribes and groups who have been in certain geographic regions longer than modern civilization. Regional recipes like Polynesian poi, made from the taro root; the nopalitos of the Southwestern United States, made from prickly pear cactus; the pounded yam bread of Africa; or the acorn mush of North America are all derived from an abundant plant in the area. These recipes are also fairly simple, so it's likely that people in these regions were eating the same food well before agriculture and the Cuisinart.

These staple foods are a great indication of how hunter/gatherers ate on a regular basis and it is recommended that you make and eat the cuisine from indigenous ingredients where ever you live or travel. Doing so helps to edify about different cultures and lends insight into the effort it takes to procure sustenance. When you complete the process that's required to make acorn mush, for instance, you'll have more of an appreciation for other foods and perhaps come to realize the full value of food in general. The process involves gathering the acorns and cracking and removing the shells, then grinding them into a flour. The flour is then rinsed through, often multiple times, to remove the bitter taste, then mixed with water and hot rocks in order to cook the flour.

At this point, the acorn mush could be used for patties, bread, or soup.

Poi, nopalitos, yam bread, and acorn mush are not the most delicious foods known to man—poi is about as bland as its light purple color and wild prickly pear fruit and yams aren't ice cream sundaes either—but if the alternative were starvation, they would taste like paradise.

If you're interested in finding out what foods can be derived from the indigenous plants in your area, please reference the brief list below or visit a local state or national park. The rangers at the park should be aware of the edible plant species in the area and what the people who live off of the land make from those ingredients. There are a couple of things to note, however, when considering eating off the land:

(1) If you want to eat something found in nature, be sure to identify it exactly before trying it. Many plant species are poisonous and will cause extreme injury or even death if consumed. If you are unsure of a plant species, but would like to try it, follow the steps of the Universal Edibility Test found in the appendix.

(2) State and national parks are nature preserves and their rules and regulations must be observed to maintain a natural setting. Most park rangers will instruct you to leave the park as you found it (i.e. no extracurricular gardening).

(3) Selecting wild plants to eat usually means that pesticides are not used, which is good, but also means that there may be unwanted insects or arachnids in or around the plant. When you're looking for wild plants to bite into, make sure there's not something there that wants to bite into you first.

With those guidelines in mind, venture out to see what you can find for food in the wild. Just identifying the local edible plants can be insightful and fun. A walk on some trails in the desert-like canyon near my house alerted me to at least four different edible plants in the area: prickly pear cactus, cattails (probably not indigenous), agave, and the acacia plant. I only tried the prickly pear fruit, which was bitter, however fairly palatable; but it's good to know that there are other plants species in the nearby area that I could use in case of an emergency. The process of procuring the minimal nutrients from the prickly pears also made me more grateful for the amount of food I had stored away in my pantry at home. A backpacking site (http://www.the-ultralight-site.com/edible-plants.html) is a great resource for learning about wild plants to eat, as is the US Army's Survival Guide, which can be found on the Evolution Diet's website (http://www.evolution-diet.com/live_off_the_land. html). I've included a number of the edible plant species here with their respective Energy Indexes and Protein Indexes.

Temperate Zone Plants

Apple

Description and Habitat: Most wild apples look enough like domestic apples that the survivor can easily recognize them. Wild apple varieties are much smaller than cultivated kinds; the largest kinds usually do not exceed 5 to 7.5 centimeters in diameter, and most often less. They have small, alternate, simple leaves and often have thorns. Their flowers are white or pink and their fruits reddish or yellowish. They are found in the savanna regions of the tropics. In temperate areas, wild apple varieties are found mainly in forested areas. Most frequently, they are found on the edge of woods or in fields. They are found throughout the Northern Hemisphere.

Edible Parts: Prepare wild apples for eating in the same manner as cultivated kinds. Eat them fresh, when ripe, or cooked. Should you need to store food, cut the apples into thin slices and dry them. They are a good source of vitamins.

CAUTION: Apple seeds contain cyanide compounds. Do not eat.

Energy Index: 4.392 Protein Index: -4.291

Asparagus

Description and Habitat: The spring growth of this plant resembles a cluster of green fingers. (It looks just like the asparagus bundles you find in the supermarket) The mature plant has fern-like, wispy foliage and red berries. Its flowers are small and greenish in color. Several species have sharp, thorn like structures. Asparagus is found worldwide in temperate areas. Look for it in fields, old home sites, and fence rows.

Edible Parts: Eat the young stems before leaves form. Steam or boil them for 10 to 15 minutes before eating. Raw asparagus may cause nausea or diarrhea. The fleshy roots are a good source of starch.

WARNING: Do not eat the asparagus fruits of any kind since some are toxic.

Energy Index: 0.784 Protein Index: 0.799

Beechnut

Description and Habitat: Beech trees are large (9 to 24 meters tall), symmetrical forest trees that have smooth, light-gray bark and dark green foliage. The character of its bark plus its clusters of prickly seedpods, clearly distinguish the beech tree in the field. This tree is found in the Temperate Zone. It

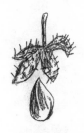

Beechnut

grows wild in the eastern United States, Europe, Asia, and North Africa. It is found in moist areas, mainly in the forests. This tree is common throughout southeastern Europe and across temperate Asia. Beech relatives are also found in Chile, New Guinea, and New Zealand.

Edible Parts: The mature beechnuts readily fall out of the husk like seedpods. You can eat these dark brown triangular nuts by breaking the thin shell with your fingernail and removing the white, sweet kernel inside. Beechnuts are one of the most delicious of all wild nuts. They are a most useful survival food because of the kernel's high oil content.

You can also use the beechnuts as a coffee substitute. Roast them so that the kernel becomes golden brown and quite hard. Then pulverize the kernel and, after boiling or steeping in hot water, you have a passable coffee substitute.

Energy Index: 5.52 Protein Index: -4.061

Blackberries

Description and Habitat: These plants have prickly stems (canes) that grow upward, arching back toward the ground. They have alternate, usually compound leaves. Their fruits may be red, black, yellow, or orange. These plants grow in open, sunny areas at the margin of woods, lakes, streams, and roads throughout temperate regions. The blackberry plant is a weed, so it grows and grows and doesn't stop (Settlers brought the plant into Yosemite valley in the 1800s because they knew it would grow steadily, much to the bane of modern conservationists). In the Pacific North West, you'll be able to spot blackberries everywhere during the summer. There is also an arctic raspberry.

Edible Parts: The fruits and peeled young shoots are edible. Flavor varies greatly—darker fruit usually means sweeter.

Energy Index: 1.266 Protein Index: -0.552

Blueberries

Description and Habitat: These shrubs vary in size from 30 centimeters to 3.7 meters tall. All have alternate, simple leaves. Their fruits may be dark blue, black, or red and have many small seeds. These plants prefer open, sunny areas. They are found throughout much of the north temperate regions and at higher elevations in Central America.

Edible Parts: Their fruits are edible when raw.

Energy Index: 4.207 Protein Index: -3.897

Burdock

Description and Habitat: This green plant has wavy-edged, arrow-shaped leaves and flower heads in bur-like clusters. It grows up to 2 meters tall, with purple or pink flowers and a large, fleshy root. Burdock is found worldwide in the North Temperate Zone. Look for it in open waste areas during the spring and summer.

Edible Parts: Peel the tender leaf stalks and eat them raw or cook them like other greens. The roots are also edible boiled or baked.

Energy Index: 1.357 Protein Index: -0.800

Cranberry

Description and Habitat: This plant has tiny leaves arranged alternately. Its stem creeps along the ground. Its fruits are red berries. (They look just like the domestic ones). It only grows in open, sunny, wet areas in the colder regions of the Northern Hemisphere.

Edible Parts: The berries are very tart when eaten raw. Cook in a small amount of water and add sugar, if available, to make a jelly.

(With sugar as jelly) Energy Index: 16.558 Protein Index: -16.514

Dandelion

Description and Habitat: Dandelion leaves have a jagged edge, grow close to the ground, and are seldom more than 20 centimeters long. Its flowers are bright yellow. There are several dandelion species. Dandelions grow in open, sunny locations throughout the Northern Hemisphere.

Edible Parts: All parts are edible. Eat the leaves raw or cooked. Boil the roots as a vegetable. Roots roasted and ground are a good coffee substitute. Dandelions are high in vitamins A and C and in calcium.

Energy Index: 1.719 Protein Index: -0.304

Fireweed

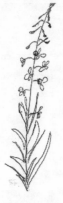

Fireweed

Description and Habitat: This plant grows up to 1.8 meters tall. It has large, showy, pink flowers and lance-shaped leaves. Its relative, the dwarf fireweed (Epilobium latifolium), grows 30 to 60 centimeters tall. Tall fireweed is found in open woods, on hillsides, on stream banks, and near seashores in arctic regions. It is especially abundant in burned-over areas.

Dwarf fireweed is found along streams, sandbars, and lakeshores and on alpine and arctic slopes.

Edible Parts: The leaves, stems, and flowers are edible in the spring but become tough in summer. You can split open the stems of old plants and eat the pith raw.

Energy Index: 0.042 Protein Index: 1.600

Grapes

Description and Habitat: The wild grape vine climbs with the aid of tendrils. Most grape vines produce deeply lobed leaves similar to the cultivated grape. Wild grapes grow in pyramidal, hanging bunches and are black-blue to amber, or white when ripe. Wild grapes are distributed worldwide. Some kinds are found in deserts, others in temperate forests, and others in tropical areas. Wild grapes are commonly found throughout the eastern United States as well as in the southwestern desert areas. Most kinds are rampant climbers over other vegetation. The best place to look for wild grapes is on the edges of forested areas. Wild grapes are also found in Mexico. In the Old World, wild grapes are found from the Mediterranean region eastward through Asia, the East Indies, and to Australia. Africa also has several kinds of wild grapes.

Edible Parts: The ripe grape is the portion eaten. Grapes are rich in natural sugars and, for this reason, are much sought after as a source of energy-giving wild food. None are poisonous.

Energy Index: 7.124 Protein Index: -6.884

Hazelnuts

Description and Habitat: Hazelnuts grow on bushes 1.8 to 3.6 meters high. One species in Turkey and another in China are large trees. The nut itself grows in a very bristly husk that conspicuously contracts above the nut into a long neck. The different species vary in this respect as to size and shape. Hazelnuts are found over wide areas in the United States, especially the eastern half of the country and along the Pacific coast. These nuts are also found in Europe where they are known as filberts. The hazelnut is common in Asia, especially in eastern Asia from the Himalayas to China and Japan. The hazelnut usually grows in the dense thickets along stream banks and open places. They are not plants of the dense forest.

Edible Parts: Hazelnuts ripen in the autumn when you can crack them open and eat the kernel. The dried nut is extremely delicious. The nut's high oil content makes it a good survival food. In the unripe stage, you can crack them open and eat the fresh kernel. Note: this is a tree nut that may cause allergies. Eat with caution!

Energy Index: 3.654 Protein Index: 1.948

Mulberry

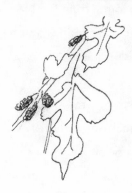

Mulberry

Description and Habitat: This tree has alternate, simple, often lobed leaves with rough surfaces. Its fruits are blue or black and many seeded. Mulberry trees are found in forests, along roadsides, and in abandoned fields in Temperate and Tropical Zones of North America, South America, Europe, Asia, and Africa.

Edible Parts: The fruit is edible raw or cooked. It can be dried for eating later.

CAUTION: When eaten in quantity, mulberry fruit acts as a laxative. Green, unripe fruit can be hallucinogenic and cause extreme nausea and cramps.

Energy Index: 3.554 Protein Index: -2.847

Oak

Description and Habitat: Oak trees have alternate leaves and acorn fruits. There are two main groups of oaks: red and white. The red oak group has leaves with bristles and smooth bark in the upper part of the tree. Red oak acorns take 2 years to mature. The white oak group has leaves without bristles and a rough bark in the upper portion of the tree. White oak acorns mature in 1 year. Oak trees are found in many habitats throughout North America, Central America, and parts of Europe and Asia.

Edible Parts: All acorns are edible, but often contain large quantities of bitter substances. White oak acorns usually have a better flavor than red oak acorns. Gather and shell the acorns. Soak red oak acorns in water for 1 to 2 days to remove the bitter substance. You can speed up this process by putting wood ashes in the water in which you soak the acorns. Boil the acorns or grind them into flour and use the flour for baking. You can use acorns that you baked until very dark as a coffee substitute.

Energy Index: 3.887 Protein Index: -2.701

Onion

Description and Habitat: Allium cernuum is an example of the many species of wild onions and garlics, all easily recognized by their distinctive odor. Wild onions and garlics are found in open, sunny areas throughout the temperate regions. Cultivated varieties are found anywhere in the world.

Edible Parts: The bulbs and young leaves are edible raw or cooked. Use in soup or to flavor meat.

CAUTION: There are several plants with onion like bulbs that are extremely poisonous. Be certain that the plant you are using is a true onion or garlic. Do not eat bulbs with no onion smell.

Energy Index: 1.998 Protein Index: -1.532

Persimmons

Description and Habitat: These trees have alternate, dark green, elliptic leaves. The flowers are inconspicuous. The fruits are orange, have a sticky consistency, and have several seeds. The persimmon is a common forest margin tree. It is widespread in Africa, eastern North America, and the Far East.

Edible Parts: The leaves are a good source of vitamin C. The fruits are edible raw or baked. To make tea, dry the leaves and soak them in hot water. You can also eat the roasted seeds.

Energy Index: 1.280 Protein Index: -1.097

Purslane

Description and Habitat: This plant grows close to the ground. It is seldom more than a few centimeters tall. Its stems and leaves are fleshy and often tinged with red. It has paddle shaped leaves, 2.5 centimeter or less long, clustered at the tips of the stems. Its flowers are yellow or pink. Its seeds are tiny and black. It grows in full sun in cultivated fields, field margins, and other weedy areas throughout the world.

Edible Parts: All parts are edible. Wash and boil the plants for a tasty vegetable or eat them raw. Use the seeds as a flour substitute or eat them raw.

Energy Index: 1.000 Protein Index: 0.034

Strawberry

Description and Habitat: Strawberry is a small plant with a three-leaved growth pattern. It has small, white flowers usually produced during the spring. Its fruit is red and fleshy. Strawberries are found in the North Temperate Zone and also in the high mountains of the southern Western Hemisphere. Strawberries prefer open, sunny areas. They are commonly planted.

Edible Parts: The fruit is edible fresh, cooked, or dried. Strawberries are a good source of vitamin C. You can also eat the plant's leaves or dry them and make a tea with them.

WARNING: Eat only white-flowering true strawberries. Other similar plants without white flowers can be poisonous.

Energy Index: 1.954 Protein Index: -1.582

Walnut

Description and Habitat: Walnuts grow on very large trees, often reaching 18 meters tall. The divided leaves characterize all walnut spades. The walnut itself has a thick outer husk that must be removed to reach the hard inner shell of the nut. The English walnut, in the wild state, is found from southeastern Europe across Asia to China and is abundant in the Himalayas. Several other species of walnut are found in China and Japan. The black walnut is common in the eastern United States.

Edible Parts: The nut kernel ripens in the autumn. You get to the walnut meat by cracking the shell. Walnut meats are highly nutritious because of their protein and oil content.

Energy Index: 5.442 Protein Index: 0.979

Tropical Zone Plants

Bamboo

Description and Habitat: Bamboo is a rapidly growing grass in the family Poaceae. Some bamboo species can grow to over 33 meters tall. Bamboo is native to China and surrounding Southeast Asian countries.

Edible Parts: The wood grows hard fast, and must be harvested while the plant is still very young (before they are two weeks old). Peel the outer layer and parboil to remove natural bitterness and woody texture.

Energy Index: 1.157 Protein Index: 0.521

Cashew

Description and Habitat: The cashew is an evergreen tree that may grow to over 15 meters tall. The trunk is twisted and gnarled and leads to a canopy of leaves. The branches support aromatic flower bunches and a fruit with the cashew nut at the end of the fruit. The cashew tree is indigenous to South America but has been brought to Asia and other tropical regions.

Edible Parts: The fruit, once ripe, can be eaten or crushed and made into jam. The nut is the most prized product of the cashew tree, but also has obstacles to its edibility. The nut is laced with a poison oak allergen urushiol, which can cause dermatitis. There is also a toxic resin inside the shell of the nut, which may spoil the inner edible portion if dealt with incorrectly.

WARNING: Do not eat cashews without steaming to release the urushiol (the same toxic chemical on poison ivy) as it may cause extreme irritation or poisoning.

Energy Index: 7.942 Protein Index: -3.004

Coconut

Description and Habitat: The long-lived coconut palm grows to 20-30 meters and has long (4-6 m) pinnate leaves. The fruit of the coconut has a large and rough brown skin.

Edible Parts: The interior of the coconut fruit contains a 4-8 cm thick fibrous meat with sugar, fiber, and protein. The milk of the fruit is also edible. An alcoholic beverage can also created from the tree's sugar sap and consumed in the opened coconut shell with a bamboo straw and palm tree umbrella.

Meat: Energy Index: 3.446 Protein Index: -2.109
Milk: Energy Index: 3.165 Protein Index: -1.691

Sugarcane

Description and Habitat: Sugarcane is a grass that grows to about 4 to 5 meters tall in just under a year, then produces a flower stalk. The stem of the grass is full of sucrose at this point and can be eaten raw, or processed to derive pure sugar. Sugarcane originated in Southeast Asia (New Guinea and Indonesia) before ancient times but can be found in most tropical zones today (2/3rds of the world's sugar production comes from sugarcane).

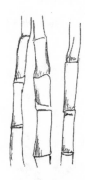

Sugarcane

Edible Parts: The inner shoots are fibrous but full of natural sugars. Crush and boil shoots to produce a molasses from the extract.

Energy Index: 7.040 Protein Index: -7.040

Taro

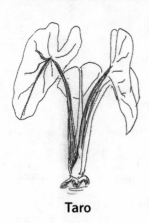

Taro

Description and Habitat: The taro plant is an herb (1-2 m tall) with large flat leaves that are connected to their stems near the center of the leaf. The plant thickens at the base and contains an underground corm. Taro is the staple food for many Pacific Island communities and parts of Southeast Asia.

Edible Parts: Wash and peel the corm, then boil to soften and rid the corm of the unpleasant needle-like crystals (oxalic acid) that exists throughout the plant. Eat like a baked potato or mash it to add to soups.

Energy Index: 0.558 Protein Index: -0.136

Desert Zone Plants

Agave

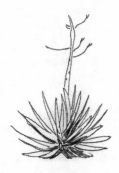

Agave

Description and Habitat: The agave plant, which can grow up to 4 meters, is an evergreen perennial with thick leaves and a tall flowering stem. Agave likes the dry and sandy soils of North American desert.

Edible Parts: The heart of the agave can be baked or soaked in water to produce a flavorful beverage. The sap from the flowering stems can be used as syrup and can be fermented to create Mescal, a potent alcoholic beverage. Agave hearts are also fermented to create tequila.

Energy Index: -0.080 Protein Index: 0.465

Amaranth

Description and Habitat: These plants, which grow 90 centimeters to 150 centimeters tall, are abundant weeds in many parts of the world. All amaranth have alternate simple leaves. They may have some red color present on the stems. They bear minute, greenish flowers in dense clusters at the top of the plants. Their seeds may be brown or black in weedy species and light-colored in domestic species. Look for amaranth along roadsides, in disturbed waste areas, or as weeds in crops throughout the world. Some amaranth species have been grown as a grain crop and a garden vegetable in various parts of the world, especially in South America.

Edible Parts: All parts are edible, but some may have sharp spines you should remove before eating. The young plants or the growing tips of older plants are an excellent vegetable. Simply boil the young plants or eat them raw. Their seeds are very nutritious. Shake the tops of older plants to get the seeds. Eat the seeds raw, boiled, ground into flour, or popped like popcorn.

Energy Index: 0.250 Protein Index: 1.549

Date Palm

Description and Habitat: The date palm is a thick-trunked tree with bushy leaves sprouting from the top. Half of the trees are male and the other are female (only females produce fruit). The date palm originated in Northern Africa, and possible Southern Asia, but has spread to North America and elsewhere.

Edible Parts: The fruit, which is known as a date, when ripe, is an extremely sweet and delicious, fibrous treat. The seed (one per date) are inedible.

Energy Index: 23.637 Protein Index: -23.347

Prickly Pear Cactus

Description and Habitat: This cactus has flat, pad like stems that are green. Many round, furry dots that contain sharp-pointed hairs cover these stems. This cactus is found in arid and semiarid regions and in dry, sandy areas of wetter regions throughout most of the United States and Central and South America. Some species are planted in arid and semiarid regions of other parts of the world.

Edible Parts: All parts of the plant are edible. Peel the fruits and eat them fresh or crush them to prepare a refreshing drink. Avoid the tiny, pointed hairs. Roast the seeds and grind them to a flour.

CAUTION: Avoid any prickly pear cactus like plant with milky sap because they are likely poisonous.

Energy Index: -0.373 Protein Index: 0.750

Kelp is another extremely healthy food that can be found in most coastal waters. Kelp is a valuable source of Iodine and vitamin C and is easy to procure and prepare.

Coastal Plants

Kelp

Description and Habitat: Commonly known as seaweed, this form of algae is an abundant and healthy food source that can be found around the world in coastal areas.

Edible Parts: All parts are edible, but the large leaves (fronds) are most usable. Eat raw or dry over a fire/oven to help keep. The dried kelp can be crushed to season other foods.

Energy Index: 0.796 Protein Index: 0.204

There are many other species of plants that can be healthy and tasty when found in the wild, but some don't have adequate nutritional information available for publishing. The U.S. Army Survival Manual lists these plants as edible as well: arrowroot, cattail, chestnut, chicory, chufa, daylily, nettle, pokeweed, sassafras, sheep sorrel, thistle, water lily and lotus, wild rose, wood sorrel, breadfruit, and acacia.

While eating off the land is a great way to get in touch with your inner hunter/gatherer, it's not worth getting sick from an accidental poisoning. There are certain guidelines that you should always follow when looking for food to eat in the wild. The U.S. Army Survival Manual says to avoid potentially poisonous plants; you should stay away from plants that have these characteristics:

- Milky or discolored sap
- Beans, bulbs, or seeds inside pods
- Bitter or soapy taste
- Spines, fine hairs, or thorns
- Dill, carrot, parsnip, or parsley-like foliage
- Almond scent in woody parts and leaves
- Grain heads with pink, purplish, or black spurs
- Three-leaved growth pattern (as in poison ivy)

With these guidelines and helpful descriptions, you will be able to develop a stronger connection to the land and identify closer to your hunter/gatherer ancestors. Living off the land can be an enjoyable and enlightening experience if the proper precautions are taken. Not to mention knowledge about living off the land could possible save your life, just ask Truman Everts.

'Tis the season

A couple months ago, a friend of mine in Chicago had lunch with a French businessman, who was in town for a meeting. The two went to a restaurant that boasted regional fare, which pleased the Frenchman. Throughout the lunch, however, my friend's acquaintance from across the pond kept chuckling and snickering in only a way that the French can get away with. When monsieur laughed at the dessert, my friend felt compelled to find out what was so funny. His lunch partner explained that much of the food that the restaurant had served wasn't from the area—and worse, a lot of the ingredients weren't even in season. How this gourmand knew all of the horticultural statistics about the area is beyond me, but I've come to learn that the French are particularly in tune with seasonal foods. If you've ever ventured to the land of crêperies and patisseries, you'll find a population obsessed with their food. It's not uncommon for each person to have a vegetable garden (a potager) or to know someone with one where fresh, seasonal produce can be acquired daily. No wonder the French region of Normandy is sometimes called the land of a thousand gardens.

What the beret-pushers know that most Americans don't is the value of fresh, in-season food. In a time of eternal shelf life and a culture of instant gratification, sticking to seasonal food is a strange concept but it is another way to ensure that you are eating the foods that you were designed to eat. When our prehistoric friends were out gathering food, they had no option to fly fresh fruit in from the other side of the world or select a ripe avocado from a greenhouse farm—everyday occurrences in what British food writer Joanna Blythman calls our *Permanent Global Summertime*. A perpetual summer may seem like a nice goal but it's not natural but there is virtue in the change of seasons. Prehistoric hunter/gatherers ate what was in season around them; and in temperate North American regions, that usually meant apricots, broccoli, spinach, and ginger in the spring; blueberries, tomatoes, green beans, and basil in the summer; apples, pears, and sweet potatoes in the fall; and leeks, potatoes, and winter squash in the winter months.

In today's Permanent Global Summertime, we can find all the above foods at the supermarket all year round—in cans or raw and having been flown in from another hemisphere; but there are numerous benefits to sticking to Natural Man's diet of eating specifically what is in season. Seasonal foods are:

(1) More nutritional. While being able to find a strawberry at the grocery in the middle of a Minnesota winter may be considered one of the 7 modern wonders of the world, it

means that the fruit was flown in from a farm a light year away and was probably picked before it was ripe, which reduces the nutritional content. Also, transportation of vegetables or fruits may mean freezing the produce, which further reduces its nutritional value. Out-of-season foods take longer to get to your grocery cart, thus they spend less time soaking up nutrients and more time in a cargo hull.

(2) Better for the environment. In addition to reducing nutritional content, transportation of food from different climates or hemispheres is also more damaging to the environment. A truck carrying corn from a nearby farm does little environmental damage compared to a few trucks and a few planes or ships that might be required to get Northerners a mango in February.

(3) Easier on the pocketbook. All of that traveling for fruits and vegetables also increases the price of the imported goods. If you're not aware of how cheap blueberries are in July when they're in season, it may not be shocking to see a small container at the store for twice as much in December, but it's always cheaper to buy something in season.

As described in Part Three, the hunter/gatherer diet was limited to natural foods, which may equate —for some people —to a monotonous menu and perhaps even insufficient vitamins and minerals at times. A skeptic might say that it's no wonder why hunter/gatherers were so fit—they were completely bored with what they had to eat. In a sense, this is true—one of the reasons why it's so easy to become overweight in today's society is that there is so much variety available to us at all times so we can eat and eat and never run out of exciting new treats. Yes, we have variety in our supermarkets, however, hunter/gatherers got a lot more out of their surroundings

than we may give them credit for and it turns out that our prede-
cessors had more of an assortment of foods in their diet than we do
today. As New York Times writer Michael Pollan explains, "Today, a mere four crops account for two-thirds of the calories humans eat." Pollan
is referring to the
staple foods: corn,
soybeans, wheat,
rice. "When you
consider that hu-
mankind has his-

 An Evolution Diet Essential

Eating produce and meats that are in season
is healthier, less expensive, and better for
the environment.

torically consumed some 80,000 edible species, and that 3,000 of
these have been in widespread use, this represents a radical simpli-
fication of the food web." While eating only what's in season may
seem limiting, eating like our prehistoric ancestors actually opens
up the menu to hundreds of foods that aren't typically consumed.

The diet variety for hunter/gatherers applies to animal
food as well as plant food. Of course, much of the animal food that
our ancestors ate (e.g. grasshoppers) would gross out the average
Safeway shopper today, but greater variety in food selection leads
to better nutrition. It also helps if the animals we eat are wild as opposed to being farm-raised and fed the same four grains that make
up the rest of our diet. Bruce Watkins of the Center for Enhancing
Foods to Protect Health at Purdue University has found that wild
game such as deer, elk, and bison have a better omega-3 to omega-
6 ratio. And this is not to mention a substantial source of protein
for our hunter/gatherer friends as well as many modern cultures:
insects, which, according to the Entomological Society of America,
are more nutritious and have more minerals than standard lean
beef. Besides bugs, which have short life spans and are unavail-
able during the colder months of the year, most animals don't have

seasons and are available all year round—a notable exception is fish, some of which migrate according to water temperatures and reproductive routines.

While benefits to eating what's in season are seemingly endless, there is one concern that we should consider before adhering to a seasonal and local food diet. We are used to getting certain vitamins from our favorite foods throughout the year, but if that particular food isn't available 3/4ths of the year, we might have to find another compensatory food to maintain our vitamin intake. As seen in the chart below, each season has plenty of healthy, vitamin-filled fresh foods, but if there is something missing in your diet, a complete multivitamin could be beneficial. To appraise your current diet and to find out if you're deficient in any essential component of your diet, we suggest you log your diet on the free Evolution Diet Health Tracker (found here: http://www.evolution-diet.com/health_tracker.htm). Once you've registered and entered your daily intake and quantity, click on 'Save and Analyze'. The link to 'Calculate Nutrient Intakes from Foods' will allow you to assess your need for additional nutrients and perhaps a multivitamin supplement. While most people's diets will fluctuate from day to day, you should be in the general range for the recommendations on that page and should be able to determine your need for any supplement.

If you're lacking in some areas, a multivitamin may be a good, inexpensive option. Most multivitamins have similar components and are produced in FDA-registered facilities, but don't be fooled by price. A good multivitamin should cost no more than $0.10 a day. We offer our own top-of-the-line multivitamin (found at http://www.evolution-diet.com/multivitamin.html) for exactly that. One should be able to get all of the vitamins and minerals recommended daily with a diet including vegetables, fruits and fish, but cost and availability may make a multivitamin extremely valuable. With vitamin and mineral concerns covered, we can focus on all the other previously mentioned benefits of eating foods that are in season.

Spring

Apricots, Artichokes, Asparagus, Avocados, Basil, Beans, Beets, Berries, Broccoli, Brussels Sprouts, Cabbage, Chinese Cabbage, Cucumbers, Ginger, Radish Head or Iceberg Lettuce, Mangoes, New Potatoes, Okra, Sweet Oranges, Papayas, Peas, Pineapple, Chile Peppers Sweet Peppers, Rhubarb, Shallots, Spinach, Strawberries, Sugar Snap Peas, Summer Squash, Turnips

Summer

Avocados, Apricots, Basil, Beans, Beets, Berries, Cherries, Corn, Cucumbers, Dates, Eggplant, Figs, Grapes, Green Beans, Mangoes, Melons, Okra, Peaches, Chile Peppers, Shell Beans, Sweet Peppers, Plums, Summer Squash, Tomatoes, Watermelon

Autumn

Apples, Beets, Broccoli, Brussels Sprouts, Cabbage, Chinese Cabbage, Cauliflower, Celery Root, Chicory, Cranberries, Cucumbers, Dates, Fennel, Grapes, Greens, Head or Iceberg Lettuce, Leaf Lettuce, Mushrooms, Nuts, Okra, Mandarin, Oranges, Pears, Chile Peppers, Sweet Peppers, Persimmons, Pomegranates, Pumpkins, Quince, Rutabagas, Shallots, Spinach, Winter Squash, Star Fruit, Sweet Potatoes

Winter

Avocados, Broccoli, Brussels Sprouts, Cabbage, Chinese Cabbage, Cauliflower, Celery Root, Chicory, Fennel, Grapefruit, Greens, Leeks, Wild Mushrooms, Mandarin Oranges, Minneola Tangelos, Sweet Oranges, Papayas, Potatoes, Pears, Spinach, Sweet Potatoes, Winter Squash

Part Nine
Liquid of Life
(The Importance of Water)

"Water is the most neglected nutrient in your diet but one of the most vital."

- Kelly Barton

One nutrient that was not appropriately emphasized in the first edition of *The Evolution Diet* is water. The crucial fluid, which makes up most of our body and weight, is vital to optimal health and especially important when trying to get to an ideal weight. As mentioned in the Introduction, when gimmick diets claim that you can lose 20 pounds in one week, it could very well be true, but the weight won't be in fat, it will be in water, which you need considerably more than fat for optimal health.

Permit me to do the math on this: 20 pounds of unwanted fat at 3,500 calories a pound is 70,000 calories of stored energy. For someone to burn that many calories in one week means they would have to run for 9 hours straight at 5 miles an hour, each day and tack those burned calories on to their usual basal metabolic rate. Double marathon for seven straight days, anyone?

If someone were to lose 20 pounds in a week on such a diet, it would mostly be in water weight, which means he or she would be producing one of the worst situations possible: the unhealthy fat the dieter was trying to lose would still be lurking around the love handles, and the quintessential nutrient, water, would be depleted. We all know the dangers of having too much body weight in fat (too much fat leads to heart conditions and diabetes among other problems), but many don't realize the problems associated with too little water. Chronic dehydration does a number of nasty things to the thirsty person including elevating whole blood viscosity, plasma viscosity, hematocrit, and fibrinogen in the blood, which all contribute to the number one killer in America, coronary heart disease.

For those who are trying to lose fat, a process that adds additional stress to the cardiovascular system, losing water also is one of the worst things they can do. If you want to lose weight, you *can* do it, but you can do it by eating foods when they should be eaten, avoiding Artificially Extreme Foods, elevating and maintaining a consistent basal metabolism, exercising more, and other healthy methods, not by reducing water intake.

In fact, dehydration not only decreases cardiovascular health, it also inhibits the metabolism of fat. Without a sufficient supply of water in the body, one's renal system cuts back on its filtering duties, outsourcing them to the liver. With an additional workload from the kidneys, the liver can't do one of its main jobs, metabolizing fat for energy. This results in more stored fat, compounding the already stressful situation. Getting thirsty anyone?

Suffice it to say, a healthy amount of water in one's diet is extremely important. So, how much is a healthy amount? The generally accepted rule of thumb is eight 8-ounce glasses a day.

This changes, naturally, the more active you are, the dryer the air is around you, the taller you are, or the more weight you have. The International Sports Medicine Institute has developed a better gauge of ½ ounce of water per pound of body weight per day. This means a person weighing 160 pounds should drink *ten* 8-ounce glasses a day.

Along with a more consistent metabolism, better cardio-vascular health and other benefits, an increase in water intake will also satisfy your hunger longer without adding calories. It's true that for some, water doesn't have the same appeal as a 64 oz. Big Gulp full of Mountain Dew, but to fully benefit from H_2O, it's important to drink it without the added carbonation and sugar found in a soft drink.

We can get our needed water from various sources, including our fruits and vegetables, which can be up to 96 percent water as is the case with squash, nuts (almonds are about 7 percent water), and, of course, beverages. Drinking-water is extremely abundant in our society today: we can get it at the tap if you don't mind a few extra minerals and chemicals; get it from the mountain stream, as some bottled water brands purport; from the ocean through desalinization; or from a factory that purifies water. With all these sources, it's difficult to make an excuse for not getting enough water.

Natural Thirst

With most of our drinking water coming from man-made sources instead of natural locations (the faucet as opposed to the local freshwater spring), it may strike you as unnatural that we drink so much of it or that it is so abundant. Surely, Nat couldn't go to his local Paleolithic mini-mart and pick up a week's supply of reverse-osmosis water in convenient 16-ounce bottles. Is it possible that water in today's society could be one of the Artificially Extreme Foods we should avoid in our diets? Could it be that the current push for more water in our diet is just a great marketing ploy to get us unwitting consumers to buy a $2 bottle of one of the most plentiful nutrients on Earth? Well, while the *price* of water at the grocery store may very well be *unnatural*, the fact that we drink so much of it isn't. In fact, Natural Man was probably more well-hydrated than we are today, even without our Culligan man and our Dasani bottlers. Marvin Harris, author of *Our Kind* says that humans' thirst for water has only played a major role in our cultural lives recently. According to him, hunter/gatherers stayed relatively close to fresh water as a general rule and only in the last few hundred years have large populations ventured into the arid lands that make water a valuable commodity. Harris says that water, "was not the kind of stuff for which people would exchange food and services." If you offered Nat a bottle of Arrowhead or Dasani and tried to get two *bones* for it, he would laugh at you. Why would he trade something of value for water, which is everywhere?

This is not to diminish the value of water to Nat's physiology. He needed water back in his day as much as we need it today, it was just more plentiful for him. Nat was drinking constantly from streams, fresh snow, lakes, and getting a good deal of water from his food.

That may have been true for residents of lush, high-rainfall areas, but what of the hunter/gatherers in desert environs like the aborigines of Western Australia? Aren't they adapted to live without 64 ounces of abmba (Aboriginal word for water)? One would think that the climate in which these hunter/gatherers find themselves, which is exceptionally dry with rare and inconsistent rainfall and extremely high evaporation rate, would mean that they are designed to work on much less water than their counterparts in rainier places. It turns out, though, that Aborigines aren't adapted for less water, they're just really good at finding the water that is out there.

Early European explorers in Australia were amazed by the ability of such seemingly primitive peoples to find waterholes without any scientific equipment. Faced with a daunting task of staying hydrated on his Western Australian journeys, Lawrence Wells, an Australian explorer, wrote in 1899 that, "...without [an Aborigine] guide in such a country one is almost powerless." It was the Aborigines who, mainly through rote memorization, knew where the water holes were located. The hunter/gatherers would capitalize on small, inconsistent water holes when they were filled after a rain, then return to larger, more consistent holes when the smaller ones had dried up.

Aborigines were also able to find water in unlikely places like tree stumps, tree roots, man-made dams, and, believe it or not, frogs (the water-holding frog *Cyclorana* platycephala to be specific). So, while the Aborigines lived in an inhospitable climate, they still needed water and were able to find it in creative ways. So, it is evident that even the most well acclimated humans still need water, and we're no different.

Part Ten

How Not to Eat
(From Atkins to The Zone)

"Inside me lives a this gal just crying to get out, but I can usually just shut her up with cookies..."

-Anonymous

Since the first trial dieters began the Evolution Diet, a new wave of diets have taken over the zeitgeist, knocking popular books like *Dr. Atkins New Diet Revolution* by Atkins and *The New Cabbage Soup Diet* by Danbrot down a few notches on the bestseller list. As I described in the Introduction, fad diets are as ubiquitous as they are unhelpful, but some can be fairly humorous. There's the Russian Air Force Diet, which basically consists of coffee in the morning and meat for the rest of the day. As Faddiet.com states, "sure they lost the cold war, but they looked good doing it." There's also the Grapefruit Diet, which promotes the bittersweet citrus fruit in every meal and was no doubt thought up by the Ruby Red Council of America. There's the Chicken Soup Diet, the Peanut Butter Diet, the Applesauce Diet and the Chocolate Diet (how can "The Evolution Diet" compare with those?).

What replaced ultra-fad diets like Atkins have been a lot more common sense approaches to eating and weight loss. Instead of buying into gimmicky concepts like no-carbs or only one specific vegetable, consumers are looking into getting a well-rounded diet in a way that matches how they were designed to eat. Since the first publication of *The Evolution Diet* there has been some great information on the popular bookshelf, most notably a bestseller by Mehmet C. Oz and Michael F. Roizen, *You: On a Diet*. Roizen and Oz put together an entertaining review of the human digestive system and a collection of techniques to help people lose weight a healthy way. Much of the material reflects concepts that I came to as well, while researching for *The Evolution Diet*, such as keeping metabolism up through snacking; the differentiation of good and bad stress and its effects on weight; benefits of exercise; and briefly what our ancestors ate. But *You: On a Diet* also contains some great new ideas and concepts. The authors describe some scientific studies and offer some self-tests to get into how our bodies work and how we should be eating while bringing up some great points mixed with humorous metaphors and one liners.

You does lack a few major concepts, most notably, *when* to eat certain foods, a topic that another popular diet-book author, Jorge Cruise, covers adequately in *The 3-Hour Diet*. Cruise promotes exercise much more than the good doctors of *You* and also takes time to debunk the no-carb myth.

There has also been quite a bit of material put together about a central theme of this book, what we should eat to match the way we were designed. Admittedly, much of the material was out before the first edition of this book was released, though the ideas were arrived at independently.

The Paleo Diet, by Loren Cordain is an interesting book about, "Eating the food you were designed to eat." After seeing this subtitle, I was a little disheartened to come to the realization that the ideas I came up with weren't as original as I had first thought. I then became encouraged by what I found: truly healthy eating, in conjunction with exercise was becoming more popular. In contrast to the Atkins plan, which was extremely popular the time of the first printing of this book, *The Paleo Diet* focuses on lean, healthy meats and promotes a wealth of healthy vegetables and fruits. The main focus here is on eating natural foods, ones that our friend Nat would be able to find in his natural surroundings.

Along the same lines is Philip Goscienski's *Health Secrets of the Stone Age*, which is a thoroughly enjoyable and insightful book about the way Paleolithic man hunted, gathered, ate, and enjoyed healthy lives. *Health Secrets* is chalk full of interesting perspectives on our culture and contrasts between what we put on our plates nowadays and what our ancestors ate. The book also promotes healthy exercise and even includes a brief exercise manual with images.

While these books do describe a perfectly healthy diet, and in the case of Goscienski's book, a perfectly healthy lifestyle, The Evolution Diet distinguishes itself in a two key ways. *Paleo* stresses natural foods that a Stone Age person could only find while taking a stroll through Stonehenge or on his way to painting class in the Lascaux Cave, but for us to emulate that diet, we would be restricting our diet to a plan that lacks good health as much as it does variety. To be sure, Cordain doesn't recommend limiting one's diet to any regional fare — as described in Part Four, this would lead to an extremely repetitive and dull diet, not to mention, one that is not as healthy as we could maintain with the current wealth of our society. In this way, Cordain promotes a variety of foods, all natural, but not necessarily accessible to a pre-agriculture hunter/gatherer.

The Evolution Diet: All-Natural and Allergy Free goes further and explains how to eat those healthy foods. It wouldn't do much good to eat all the perfectly healthy foods that our ancestors ate, but eat them in such a way as to reduce the health benefits. As explained in Part Four, when LoS Hi-Fi foods are eaten with high-protein foods (potatoes with your rack of lamb), the digestion of either food is stifled. Appropriation of one's diet is just as important as food selection in attempting to eat the way we were designed.

Another distinction is that *The Paleo Diet* urges us to eat exactly in the manner of our Stone Age relatives without adapting to modern technology and the author even contradicts that. Cordain includes some foods, possibly unwittingly, that would not be found on Nat's à la carte menu. For instance, the high-fiber, high-vitamin and high-mineral food, almond (described in Part Five), which is promoted throughout *Paleo*, was not available to eat in the Paleolithic Age. As Jared Diamond describes *in Guns, Germs, and Steel*, almonds found in nature have a high level of the bitter chemical amygdalin, which easily breaks down into harmful cyanide in our digestive systems. In fact, a couple of wild, bitter almonds can *kill* a person. But, sweet almonds that have been cultivated and procured since agriculture arose are safe and, moreover, extremely healthy.

 An Evolution Diet Essential

The Evolution Diet promotes healthy foods that were around in the time of prehistoric man as well as those that have become available since.

Broccoli is another example of an extremely healthy and beneficial food that matches what we are designed to eat, but wasn't around before agriculture. The story of this cruciferous plant goes back to the early Etruscans, who came to Italy from

Asia Minor. Their cultivation of various cabbages eventually led to broccoli, which became wildly popular in the Roman Empire and ultimately the world. It seems that to say flatly that we should only eat what cavemen ate is a bit shortsighted. The point isn't to eat only what was available pre-agriculture—that would be nearly impossible—or ignore the benefits of living in a modern age; the point is to match what we were physiologically designed to eat with all the healthy and nutritious selections available today.

The Evolution Diet: All-Natural and Allergy Free does just that; it promotes all foods that were around pre-agriculture as in *Paleo*, but it doesn't exclude foods all the foods that have become available to us since, including healthy, but also slightly processed foods. It may be clear to the reader that, besides almonds and broccoli, there are a number of extremely healthy foods that weren't available to Nat in his Stone Age life, including deep-sea albacore tuna (off the coast for most of the year), chicken (an obscure bird), spinach (only recently propagated), and much more. Indeed, most of the foods we eat today hardly resemble the species that our ancestors nibbled on, which were much smaller and sometimes a less nutritious variety in some ways.

Does that throw out the entire concept of eating like we were designed to eat? No, because we can still base our diet on what our physiology expects, especially with regard to macronutrients like carbohydrates, protein, and fat, and enhance our eating experience and health with more micronutrients (vitamins and minerals) through more variety.

The basic rule of thumb is to eat natural foods. As one pundit said, never eat foods that begin with a capital letter (meaning man-made processed foods with man-made names). Unfortunately, some all-natural foods can also be unhealthy to an extent, as we saw in the section on Artificially Extreme Foods. Orange juice, while usually all-natural, is like a shot of glucose straight to the bloodstream when consumed. This all-natural beverage should be avoided in large amounts outside of heavy exercise. The basic guideline to follow is all-natural foods, but not in extreme amounts or densities.

Part Eleven
Other Factors
(What Else Can Play A Part In Your Health)

"An old friend of mine said she lost 28 pounds just by skipping every day. She skipped dessert, she skipped the candy bar after lunch, she skipped the pancakes..."

-Anonymous

"I keep trying to lose weight... but it keeps finding me!"

-Anonymous

In 2007, one of our Evolution trial dieters was making great strides in her eating habits—she was snacking on healthy, natural LoS Hi-Fi foods throughout the day and exercising regularly before a fair-sized high-protein meal almost every day. She was getting her health back in order, but she was not losing weight and she was still having trouble sleeping and this was really beginning to stress her out, which inevitably led to worse sleeping patterns. Unfortunately, food consumption wasn't the only thing this trial dieter needed to focus on. There are other factors involved in ideal health—influenced by one's diet, but not completely dependent on nutritional intake. In our trial dieter's case, the problem that was causing so much stress was stress itself. She was worrying herself into bad health. In matters concerning weight loss and energy maintenance, the food you put into your system is the number one factor, but there are other things that work with and against your diet to affect your health, including your metabolism, sleep, and stress levels. I will go over each and how it relates to the diet here.

Basal Metabolism

Everyone needs a certain amount of calories in their diet simply to live. Outside of exercise or physical activity, we need this basic level of energy to just keep our vital organs humming. The basic functions of life (e.g. breathing, circulating blood, producing body heat, etc.) actually take up the largest portion of the average person's energy output. These basic functions are called basal metabolism. The basal metabolic rate, or BMR, is the amount of energy those functions consume while at rest in room temperature (68 degrees Fahrenheit).

There are many factors that play into your BMR at any given time—how tall you are, how much you weigh, what kind of exercise you're used to, and your age among other factors. There are other important factors like amount of muscle mass, but they are very difficult to determine without sophisticated equipment. The most accurate way to determine your BMR is to measure the exchange of oxygen and carbon dioxide through your lungs. This process shows what you're taking in to fuel your cells and what you're getting rid of. A simpler method to determine your BMR is with this equation called the Harris-Benedict formula:

Adult male BMR: 66 + (6.3 x body weight in lbs.) + (12.9 x   height in inches) - (6.8 x age in years)

Adult female BMR: 655 + (4.3 x weight in lbs.) + (4.7 x height in inches) - (4.7 x age in years)

The free online health assessment on this book's companion website, http://www.evolution-diet.com, will report your BMR as well as other information like your Body Mass Index and overall HealthScore. When you get to the website, click on the link "What's Your HealthScore?" to be directed to the free resource.

Determining your BMR is a great way to gauge how much you should be eating in the span of one day, whether you want to maintain your weight or lose a couple pounds. Disregarding physical activity, you should only be eating the calories represented by your BMR if you want to maintain your weight. Calories burned from exercise (see chart in Part Twelve) can then be added to your BMR to determine how many calories you burn in a particular day. Using that number and your weight goals, you should be able to determine whether you can afford that slice of chocolate cake after your 20-minute walk.

The generally accepted average for caloric intake is 2000, which is the standard for the Recommended Daily Allowance. But you may find that you do not need to be eating that much, or you may realize you need to be eating more to compensate for your high energy expenditures per day.

Basal metabolism is extremely important to your weight because it is by far the highest calorie burner working for you. The Evolution Diet is designed to keep your metabolism going at a steady pace, and thus burn *more* calories than you may be doing right now with an unstable metabolism, which speeds up and slows down throughout the day. The process of fasting, then eating large meals throughout the day creates a rollercoaster effect for your metabolism, but when you eat the LoS Hi-Fi foods continuously in small amounts when you're hungry, you are keeping your metabolism up, and burning more calories.

Additionally, The Evolution Diet involves eating foods that take more energy to digest, also increasing the daily calorie expenditure. Foods like fiber and complex carbohydrates are more difficult to digest than sugars, and that's why they are more beneficial than energy contained in things like candy.

 Tips for increasing constant energy expenditure (while some of these do not effect the BMR, they all help you burn more calories without exerting much effort)

- Turn down the heat or air conditioning. Your body expends more calories in cold or hot temperatures.
- Don't binge and purge. Chronic yo-yo dieters on low calorie diets actually lower their BMR below that of their average intake.
- Choose your stress wisely. Short-term stress (exercise) increases your BMR, long-term stress (worrying about a deadline) decreases it.
- Get more muscle. Having more muscle mass increases your BMR, even when you're not using your muscles.
- Fidget. Believe it or not, people who have high levels of "spontaneous physical activity" have a significantly higher constant energy expenditure, on average.
- Exercise. When you work your cardiovascular and muscle systems, your body must "heal" them afterwards, thus increasing your BMR for up to 12 hours.
- Breathe freely. The more you hinder your breathing, the more you stifle your basal metabolism.

Exercise When Your Body Tells You To

Exercise may be one of the most important aspects to health. Although one can maintain an ideal *weight* without exercise, perfect overall health is impossible without at least a moderate amount of physical activity—the more the better. Exercise has been promoted early and often throughout history and it's no wonder: people who exercise live longer, on average, than do their couch potato counterparts. Additionally, the life they do lead is dramatically more enjoyable by being less physically straining during everyday activities and being less susceptible to illness.

As I described earlier, it is vital for people to make exercise a regular habit, however, The Evolution Diet will help no matter what the participant's physical activity consists of. The reason for this is that The Evolution Diet naturally adjusts to the participant's activity level. In other words, without exercise, The Evolution Diet restricts the participant to snacking on LoS Hi-Fi foods throughout the day. Unappealing as it may seem, without exercise, people should only eat those foods that are low in sugar, high in fiber all day—often, but in small portions. They should never gorge themselves on a high-protein meal because, in nature, that would only happen after exercise (hunting to Nat, the hunter/gatherer). Without exercise, only small quantities of protein should be eaten and it should be eaten in the snacking manner of the LoS Hi-Fi foods.

In addition, sugary foods, tasty as they are, would not be necessary if one did not exercise. Sugars tend to spike blood sugar (as discussed before) and, if not used immediately, just turn to fat. A sugary orange or bit of honey would compel Nat to fidget and become active and since he was not forced to sit behind a desk all day, Nat could react to the sugary food naturally. We modern Westerners, however, are confined to sitting on our bums for 8-12 hour stretches Monday through Friday. It would be easy to utilize the energy spike if you were prepared to exercise, but clicking on a mouse or meeting with the board won't quite utilize the energy and all of that excess sugar would go straight to the spare tire. In the meantime, the increased blood sugar might make you irritable or tense. So, exercising allows for a more dynamic diet, complete with large protein dinner, and healthy sugars in addition to the LoS Hi-Fi snacks.

 An Evolution Diet Essential

Exercising allows a more dynamic diet, complete with large protein dinners and sugars in addition to the LoS Hi-Fi foods.

The Evolution Diet provides a couple of guidelines for exercising that will help maximize the benefits of your work out.

(1) Exercise when you are slightly hungry or have a small amount of food in your stomach, not when you are full. When your body begins to work its muscles, your body automatically switches its focus from the digestive system to the muscles. Blood that would have gone to the stomach to aid in digestion goes instead to the quadriceps or triceps. This switch, involving vasoconstriction and vasodilatation of different body tissues, slows the nonessential bodily activities, and during exercise this means the digestive tract. The problem with this is that when people exercise, the stomach does not receive the blood it is used to getting for the process of digestion and cannot function properly, commonly producing the side effect of cramping. The old adage, "One shouldn't go into the pool or ocean right after eating a big meal," is valid, however, it only applies when one is exercising in water because cramping increases your risk of drowning. If water has a relaxing effect on

you, it may actually be *better* for you and your digestion to wade in the pool at that time.

Exercising while you're slightly hungry has other benefits too. If you are used to eating highly sugary foods, then being hungry before exercising may reduce your energy and motivation to exercise. If you are constantly on a sugar high, being hungry may make you hypoglycemic and weak feeling. However, if you maintain a steady intake of LoS Hi-Fi foods before exercise, your body will not be abnormally stressed without immediate sugar and you will have sustained energy for exercise.

(2) In order to lose weight, exercise when you are tired. This may seem odd, but it really works! Your body becomes tired for different reasons, one of which is low blood sugar. When you have low blood sugar and you push your body in the form of exercise, the body pulls the energy from stored sources, like fat.

You can also apply this to long-term exercising as well. After you've been physically active for a couple minutes, your body starts what's called aerobic exercise. This form of physical activity uses oxygen to break down the glucose that's stored throughout your body in places like the muscles, the liver, fatty acids, and in extreme situations like starvation, glucose can be derived from protein while exercising. This extremely complex process ends with the muscle cells producing energy (through the wonder molecule ATP).

(3) If you get a boost of energy while you are stationary at work or at the home, use it. Get up and walk to the water cooler; walk up and down a couple flights of stairs or walk around the block; clench and unclench your fists to get the blood flowing. If you don't mind looking a little silly, do some stretches in your office or do leg lifts behind your desk. Your body will reward you with a relaxed, yet not tired feeling afterward. If you use the sugars

that you eat immediately when they come in, you will stress your endocrine system less. Also, by doing physical activity when you get a boost of blood sugar, you will not retain all of the excess, unused energy as fat.

The Origin of Exercise

Natural Man did not exercise in the sense that we now know it today. Nat obviously didn't have an elliptical machine back in his day, nor did his pre-agriculture friends go to their local gym and lift stones every day after gathering food and painting on caves, yet they were physically fit. Their form of exercise was walking from camp to camp as they followed their food sources of plants and animals, as well as hunting when they came upon wild game.

Besides the physically active games they participated in, they were continuously moving around to get fresh picks of nuts, berries, and plants that were the staple of their diets. Then, when they had enough energy from their foraging, they would set off on major hunting expeditions, running for miles or sprinting, then attacking their prey (buffalo, deer, woolly mammoths, etc.). The attack usually consisted of spear throwing and/or wrestling, with the necessary butchering of the animal before it was consumed. It was the ability to run long distances, though, which was the differential advantage that humans had over all the other animals. Anthropologist David Carrier postulated in 1984 that early hominids used their newfound bipedalism for persistence hunting in which our ancestors would run down prey until it died from exhaustion. Carrier maintains that this hunting behavior was integral to human development and precisely how we got to a superior position in the predatory hierarchy.

This physical activity was a part of the lifestyle of all pre-historic people, not just the *man of the cave*. While women are not designed for specific hunting activities like men (modern track and field records for both sexes show a 9-20 percent difference between men and women due to their muscle and fat composition), they still were extremely active. As any handpicking farmer or garden-worker would attest, the gathering half of hunting and gathering is no cakewalk and requires sustained physical effort.

Stone Age peoples weren't off the exercise hook if they lived on the coast either. When Nat visited his cousins on the coast, they would take spears out to the lake or the ocean and, in a physically exhaustive procedure, fish for their meals.

The reward for all of this physical activity, for them, was mass quantities of highly nutritious meat. Today, whether we acknowledge it or not, we emulate the act of hunting by exercising, and in our modern world, we should only eat mass quantities of meat when we deserve it—that is, we should only eat meat after physical activity or exercise.

The Importance of Exercise

The supermodel Naomi Campbell has been quoted as saying, "I never diet. I smoke. I drink now and then. I never work out." And she is, "worth every cent." as she puts it. This quote may hit on a sentiment felt by many people: some people are just born good-looking and others are less fortunate. Naomi may have been telling the truth, but to imply that just because someone is at or below their ideal body weight that makes them healthy is absurd. Thinness does not equate to healthfulness, even in the well-fed society that we share with Mrs. Campbell.

Although many people are thin or skinny without exercise, one cannot be truly healthy without at least a moderate amount of physical activity. This is an important aspect of life, if not culture. The Evolution Diet can benefit you even if you're not exercising, but a sedentary lifestyle does require you to limit your intake of some foods, as mentioned before.

During physical activity, the human body requires a high amount of sugars to burn. In addition, exercise tears down muscles and works the systems of the body like the cardiovascular and respiratory systems. This tearing down process requires new protein to rebuild the bodily mechanics in a healthy way.

It only stands to reason that without exercise, one doesn't need as much sugar or as much protein. If one's body could talk to them during a stretch of a couch potato marathon, it would tell them that it doesn't need so much energy or building blocks. Contrary to the three-square meal approach to eating, it is not always healthy to eat so much food during periods of extended inactivity.

As described throughout the book, every type of food serves its own special purpose, and it just so happens that a lot of the food we eat is only required when we exercise. This is why exercise is such an important part of not only The Evolution Diet, but of general health. Organizing your diet in the divisions of The Evolution Diet (snacking on LoS Hi-Fi carbs throughout the day and eating a large protein meal at night) will help you, regardless of physical activity. But eating those foods appropriately, according to the amount of exercise one does, is extremely vital for optimal health.

Breathing and Sleep

Breathing is vital to good health and, if you are trying to lose weight, it is even more important to focus on. Breathing increases the healthy components in your blood (oxygen) and decreases the unhealthy (carbon dioxide), but it also determines how fast you burn calories. When someone measures your basal metabolic rate (explained earlier), they determine how much oxygen and carbon dioxide are exchanged during breathing while you're at rest. When we exercise, we breathe more, which is a product of and an indication that we are burning more calories.

Breathing is involuntary, meaning that we breathe without thinking about it, but we can also control our breathing and in extreme cases, we can restrict our breathing intentionally or subconsciously. Apnea is a condition in which the person stops breathing for 10 seconds or longer, five to 50 times an hour. It usually happens during sleep, but can happen while awake. There are three types of sleep apnea: obstructive sleep apnea, central sleep apnea, and mixed sleep apnea. The causes may include obstructive facial features or enlarged tissues in the nose or throat, but stem mainly from factors that you can alter yourself.

Some readers may consider sleep apnea a superficial inconvenience instead of the detrimental health concern it is. If you think that "holding your breath every once in a while" is not that dangerous, you may want to reconsider. Sleep apnea contributes to coronary artery disease and high blood pressure along with uncomfortable rest. In addition, sufferers of sleep apnea may experience lower alertness in their daily lives, memory problems, personality changes, lower desire for sex, anxiety, and depression. Obviously, sleep apnea also decreases the quality of sleep, which in itself is important.

Additionally, the quality of sleep, in general, has an important effect on weight loss. David Rapoport, MD, associate professor and director of the Sleep Medicine Program at the New York University School of Medicine in New York City explained how sleep affects one's appetite in a recent interview. "One of the more interesting ideas that has been smoldering and is now gaining momentum is the appreciation of the fact that sleep and sleep disruption do remarkable things to the body—including possibly influencing our weight."

 Hinderances to normal breathing:

- Drinking alcohol affects the region of the brain that controls breathing.
- Obesity affects 70 percent of the people who suffer from sleep apnea.
- Prescription drugs for allergies, depression or anxiety also increase the risk for sleep apnea.
- Stressful situations usually force people to limit their breathing—it becomes rapid, but shallow and doesn't provide the oxygen or other benefits of deep breathing.
- Bad posture may hinder the body's ability to open up the lungs during breathing.
- Anger focuses your body's attention on the subject of your anger, not on your biorhythms—so be happy.

The reason for this is sleep's effects on the hormones leptin and ghrelin. When you don't have a good night's sleep, the body drives up the levels of ghrelin, which stimulates your appetite. It also drives down the other side of the balance, leptin, which creates fat cells from excess blood sugar and signals to the brain that you are full. So, apnea makes us feel hungry even when are full—not a good thing when we're trying to lose weight. Also, when you have a bad night's sleep, as in the case of sleep apnea, you are breathing less and thus burning fewer calories throughout the night. The result is weight gain, usually. "I've had about thirty patients who, when successfully treated for their sleep apnea were able to lose weight—possibly because they had more energy, so they were more active and they just ate less," says Michael Breus, PhD, a faculty member of the Atlanta School of Sleep Medicine and director of The Sleep Disorders Centers of Southeastern Lung Care in Atlanta.

Unfortunately, the converse is also true: if one doesn't treat sleep apnea, they may become overweight or obese, which, in turn, would contribute further to their sleep apnea. The vicious cycle stops by learning to sleep well and eating better.

Hypopnea, or slowed breathing, is also a problem that causes similar, though less extreme results as apnea. Hypopnea can easily occur as a result of stress, so take a deep breath, and read on!

Stress

Our emotions are inextricably linked to our weight. Our state of mind and the emotions it produces directly trigger certain hormones in our body to be activated. Those hormones shooting around our bodies are so powerful, they can affect many things, most notably the immune system, physical strength, memory, disease, appetite, and weight loss.

Stress is a dramatic emotion that we are bound to have throughout our lives. The interesting thing about stress is that it is good for us in the short term, but extremely bad for us in the long term. Our bodies were designed to naturally deal with fear and stress on a regular basis in order to cope with, say, bears that see us as a little talking egg roll, for instance. But when we translate that fear into long-term anxiety, the body's reactions aren't life saving, they're life-threatening.

Immediate stress caused by a barking dog produces the hormone adrenaline in our bodies. This hormone tends to speed up our regular metabolic rate, increase breathing and heart rate, and for a very short time promote weight loss. However, long-term stress (like an anxiety disorder) produces the hormone cortisol, which stores fat (usually around the abdominal region). When you complement cortisol with an unregulated cultural diet that includes Big Macs and Whoppers, the result usually is massive weight gain.

The first goal for a stressful person should be to identify the sources of stress for them. This may come from all directions in life: a sniveling boss, irritating drivers on the street, personal disorganization, nagging relatives, and much, much more.

The solution is not the many pharmaceuticals on the market. In fact, those pharmaceuticals may contribute to other problems like the aforementioned sleep apnea and eventually push your ultimate goal of ideal health further away. The solution is to determine what is stressing you out and limit it. It could be your job, your family, or too much food. Although changing jobs may seem like a drastic step just to lose a few pounds, it may be the only way you will truly cure your stress. In turn, you will live a dramatically more fulfilling life.

An even better solution is to learn how to relax in situations when your *life* is not at risk. For the vast majority of people in Western culture, this happens to be all the time. When you are focusing on your health and on what your body is telling you, you will begin to notice all the overreactions you may be experiencing that are caused by stress. Take a second right now and set an alarm clock to interrupt you at some point in the next workday. When the alarm goes off, take note of your physical state. Are your muscles tense? Are you taking full and deep breaths? Are you calm? Chances are you will not be relaxed when you catch yourself with the alarm the next day and since your life will probably not be in immediate danger then, try to relax. Find a quiet place and stretch your legs and arms or just sit peacefully to regain a calm state of being. Meditation techniques are great for instant distressing, but the ultimate goal is to continually be relaxed in everyday situations.

Another way to reduce stress is to be an optimist. Remember to keep positive and look for the good out of every situation. If something has already happened in your life and is in your past, there's no sense in worrying about it. Calmly figuring out what to do is the only way that you can overcome your obstacles.

If you don't learn to relax when you're not physically at risk, your physical health including your weight will suffer. This should be enough motivation to get you to relax about the situations in your life.

Part Twelve

You've Evolved
(What Are The Benefits?)

"The first wealth is health."

-Ralph Waldo Emerson

One of the ongoing debates in politics today is health care, which costs Americans more than any other single industry and is continuing to grow. Some estimates put healthcare at a third of the Gross Domestic Product (the nation's annual paycheck) by 2050. Hospitals alone take in nearly a trillion dollars (that's a one with twelve zeros) each year and insurance keeps going up to pay for the bill. One of major factors in the rise in health care costs is America's collective waistline, which accounts for at least a tenth of the overall health care costs.

It stands to reason then, that we could reduce the heavy cost of health care dramatically and increase the standard of living (imagine going on 30 percent more vacations or having 30 percent more house) for everyone if we could all just eat what and how we were designed to eat. Conditions that are as vastly different as arthritis, heart disease, and sleep apnea are all caused by our culturally influenced diet. It is understandable that a species that has spent 2 million years eating a certain way, and is given a completely different menu within a couple thousand years will experience some problems, but the current state of affairs is not how it has to be.

There are a number of hunter/gatherer societies still around after all these generations of modern civilization, defying modern agricultural influences. The Inuit of North America, the Aborigines of Australia, and the Pygmies and !Kung of Africa are all maintaining their numbers in defiance of much pressure from their surrounding countries and cultures. Most of the people in them are remarkably fit and healthy. Despite the fact that they have no immunizations, no sanitation, and no modern medicine, they live healthy full lives and generally have life expectancies longer than some industrialized nations.

Imagine if you take the naturally evolved diet of the hunter/gatherers and combined it with the medicine and sanitation of our modern world. You would have the healthiest lifestyle possible, and that is within the reach of all of us.

Some Initial Side Effects

To return to your natural way of eating, and thus maximum health, there are a couple negative reactions you may experience at first. When you start the Evolution Diet, you may go through a 'hump' period of less energy and mild headaches. This is the natural process of weaning yourself off of the excess sugar and processed foods. Any dramatic switch in blood sugar causes the headaches from your normal routine. If you are accustomed to having copious amounts of glucose readily available for years prior to the diet, there stands to be a mild revolt from your body when you stop supplying it.

Additionally, any diet designed to take weight off will do a number of things initially. They will cause you to retain water and actually gain water weight initially. This may also be contributed by constipation—when you're lowering your calorie intake/expenditure rate, your body will want to hold on to any food you give it.

Don't fret though! This is just the natural progress of getting healthy. Any diet that drastically reduces your weight instantly is dangerous and will not last. The Evolution Diet takes a few weeks to show in your waistline, but the positive effects are instant! Once you have become acclimated to the diet you will begin to experience true health.

Some Positive Things to Look For

If you have any of the intolerances or allergies described in Part Five, you will immediately notice the absence of all associated symptoms when you return to the natural way you were designed to eat. From the abdominal pains to poor mood, all of your food-related issues will be eliminated in a matter of weeks on The Evolution Diet: All-Natural and Allergy-Free. In the famous words of late-night infomercials, but wait, there's more! Everyone, not just those who are intolerant or allergic to certain foods, will experience innumerable benefits. Here are some positive things to look for in your newly evolved life:

High Energy: Most noticeably, you will experience a constant high level of energy throughout the day. You will not get the dramatic boosts in energy from a sugar or caffeine high and you will not get the dramatic lulls that tend to follow. You will experience the balanced energy of eating naturally.

Ideal Weight: Since you will be eating when your body tells you to and what nature tells you to, you will achieve your ideal weight. You will probably be eating more often, but you will be eating less densely concentrated foods. This should allow for a pleasurable dieting experience while you lose all those pounds!

Better Sleep: The main problem with people's physiology in today's society is due to their lack of quality sleep, and their lack of quality sleep is due to their unnatural diet. The Evolution Diet specifically is planned so that you don't give yourself mass quantities of energy before you want to go to sleep and it's designed to give you the added bonus of certain amino acids that aid in sleep. Also, you will be filling your stomach to capacity once a day (dinner); this will tell your body that it's time to rest.

Relaxation: If you are stressed or irritated often, The Evolution Diet will help you relax. The constant, balanced energy level you will get throughout the day will lead to a more relaxed, less stressed person. In addition, the better sleep you will experience will also help you become more at ease.

More Enjoyment in Eating: If you're like most Evolution Dieters, you will experience a greater joy in eating. Since you are limited in your food selection at certain times of the day (meat throughout the day, for instance), you will learn to appreciate each food type more.

Better Dental Health: The process of constantly munching on things throughout the day, as specified in the Evolution Diet causes an increase in saliva output. This has been shown in many medical tests and is promoted by the use of chewing gum as a deterrent to cavities and gingivitis.

Better Physical Performance: When you begin to eat the way you were designed to eat, you will notice a marked improvement in your physical performance. This happens because you're producing energy when your body needs it and you're exercising when you are ready, not when it is convenient in your schedule.

More Motivation to Exercise: Separating your diet into food groups designed for before and after exercise will help you motivate yourself to exercise. Of course, the energy boost of Energy Foods will help, but also, the reward system of a hearty High-Protein Meal after exercise will also give you motivation to work out.

Better Concentration: Throughout the day, you should expect to have better concentration and alertness due to the constant intake of moderate amounts of energy.

Better Immune System: When your body becomes accustomed to a consistent, natural way of eating, your immune system will benefit. All the energy that used to go to your stress-inducing diet can be concentrated on fighting off viruses and bacteria.

These benefits are great and they are immediate, but the true rewards are only seen in the long run. With The Evolution Diet, you will drastically reduce your chance of heart disease, obesity, diabetes, high blood pressure, stroke, depression, ADD (attention deficit disorder), and food allergies.

These conditions are no joke and are directly caused by one's diet. Doctors across the world are calling for better diets for the majority of people. If you choose to eat what and how you were designed, you can give yourself a better, and most likely a longer life.

A Better Life

You are on your way to becoming the person you've always wanted to be. You are going to use your body's naturally designed mechanics to work for you, not against you and you are going to live a better, healthier, and happier life for it.

The novelty of eating how our hunter/gatherer ancestors ate will wear off after a few weeks or months, but so will the pounds. And once you've gotten close to your ideal weight, you will not want to look back. The eating style will become second nature and you'll be able to fight off the urges for half a pizza at 10 P.M. or a giant-sized banana sundae right after it.

Unhealthy foods will begin to look unappetizing to you and you will relish you newfound will power. You will be able to turn down any food that's not appropriate because you'll know exactly what it does to your body and how you would feel as a result of it.

The Evolution Diet: All-Natural and Allergy Free is full of common sense and backed by clinical study after clinical study— we were designed to eat in the specific manner of the hunter/gatherer and most of us aren't doing that anymore. But we know where we came from and how our bodies treat the different foods we feed it. With the principles in this book, you can regain the diet of our prehistoric ancestors and regain their health.

You now know that you have a greater chance of living longer by following The Evolution Diet, and those extra years that you live are going to be fun-filled. You will be excited to show your new self off and you'll have a deep sense of contentment inside, knowing that you've done one of the most difficult things in today's unnatural culture: achieving optimal health.

The benefits are seemingly endless, and you're going to experience them all. You are on the way to becoming the ideal you, and all it took was a little reading and the desire to live the way you were designed to live! Congratulations, you have evolved!

Part Thirteen
Everything Else
(For Your Information)

"He who has health, has hope. And he who has hope, has everything."

- Ancient Proverb

"To wish to be well is a part of becoming well."

-Seneca

Brief Health Assessment

If you are curious about your current health status, we invite you to take this brief questionnaire. A more intensive version can be found on our website (www.evolution-diet.com) for free.

1. How often do you exercise?

a. I try to avoid exercise at all cost
b. I get out every once in a while
c. I frequently walk, but don't really work out
d. I exercise a couple times a week
e. I regularly exercise more than 30 min at a time
f. I exercise once a day for 30 minutes or more

2. Which option best describes your eating habits?

a. I eat three meals a day
b. I eat lunch and dinner, but skip breakfast
c. I snack throughout the day and eat a large dinner
d. My eating schedule is random at best
e. I often fast, then eat a large meal
f. I'm constantly eating calorically dense food

3. On average, how many ounces of non-diet soft drink do you consume a day (12 oz in normal can)?

4. How much caffeinated beverage (e.g. tea, cola, coffee) do you consume a day?

5. What sounds more appealing to for lunch?

a. Broccoli with fat free ranch dressing
b. Deep fried chimichanga burrito with guacamole
c. Small plate of mixed greens with fat-free dressing
d. Wheat crackers with salsa
e. Club sandwich with French fries and a pickle
f. A few pieces of fruit

6. When you're tired during the day, you...

a. go to sleep
b. drink a cup of coffee or energy drink
c. move around or exercise
d. rest
e. eat
f. complain

7. Which activity do you prefer most?

a. Reading
b. Watching television
c. Intense physical sports
d. Cooking / cleaning
e. Talking with friends
f. Strolling on the beach

8. Have you or would you try weight loss drugs?

a. Yes
b. No

9. Are you hungry when you wake up in the morning?

a. Yes
b. No

10. What do you usually eat for your first meal after exercise?

a. Well-balanced meal
b. All/mostly carbohydrates
c. All/mostly protein
d. I'm not hungry, even hours after I exercise
e. Lots of fast food
f. Bring on the double chocolate cake!

continued

11. How would you describe your lifestyle?

a. Very relaxed; nothing bothers me
b. Relaxed; it takes a lot to get on my nerves
c. Often relaxed, but tense sometimes
d. Tense; I often get worked up
e. Stressed; I'm always tense and often nervous
f. A nervous breakdown is imminent

12. What item would most likely be in your refrigerator?

a. Bottled water
b. 2 liter of cola
c. 6-pack of beer
d. Gallon of fruit juice
e. White wine
f. 2 liter of diet soda

13. How much alcohol do you consume on average?

a. None
b. A drink every few weeks
c. 1-2 drinks a week
d. 3-6 drinks a week
e. 7-14 drinks a week
f. Many drinks a day

14. Do you intentionally avoid hydrogenated oils and trans fats?

a. Yes
b. No

15. On average, how many ounces of water or non-caloric beverage do you consume a day?

Results

1.   a-0 b-2 c-6 d-7 e-8 f-10
2.   a-5 b-3 c-10 d-2 e-2 f-2
3.   divide ounces by 3 and subtract from 10
4.   divide ounces by 4 and subtract from 10
5.   a-9 b-1 c-10 d-7 e-5 f-8
6.   a-5 b-3 c-10 d-2 e-2 f-2
7.   a-4 b-3 c-10 d-7 e-6 f-8
8.   a-1 b-10
9.   a-5 b-1
10. a-7 b-5 c-10 d-5 e-3 f-1
11. a-10 b-8 c-6 d-4 e-3 f-1
12. a-10 b-2 c-1 d-6 e-4 f-4
13. a-10 b-9 c-8 d-7 e-5 f-1
14. a-10 b-1
15. divide ounces by 8 (limit to 10)

Add your results (including negative numbers) and compare your total with the ranges below.

120 – 145: Congratulations! You are probably healthy and should keep up the good work!
100 – 119: You are probably fairly healthy, but could use some specific alterations to your diet or exercise routine.
80 – 99: You most likely need to change your eating habits and exercise routine.
50 – 79: There are significant issues with your eating and exercise habits, which may lead to health problems.
< 49: It's likely that you are significantly unhealthier than you could be. Your eating and exercise habits may be causing considerable health damage.

Breakfast and LoS Hi-Fi foods

Your body is designed to constantly eat these low sugar, high fiber foods (or LoS Hi-Fi foods) in small portions throughout the day. From when you get hungry in the morning until you eat dinner, you should be snacking on these foods.

LoS Hi-Fi foods are a source of consistent, balanced energy with some nutrition. A constant intake of small portions keeps your metabolism going at a high rate. Too much of these foods at one time, however will stifle your metabolism, overload your system with carbohydrates and cause fat gain.

Most grains and breads have minimal nutritious value, yet other LoS Hi-Fi foods, like vegetables and fruits are vital for our health. They provide the vitamins and minerals needed for life activities.

The best foods for daytime snacking are the ones with a low energy index (below 3) and a low protein index (below 2). These maximize the benefits of the LoS Hi-Fi foods. The higher the energy or protein index of a food, the worse it is for your constant snacking.

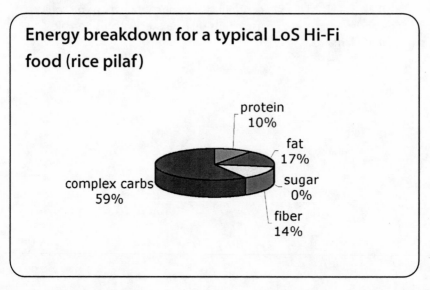

Energy breakdown for a typical LoS Hi-Fi food (rice pilaf)

protein 10%

fat 17%

complex carbs 59%

sugar 0%

fiber 14%

LoS Hi-Fi foods (In order by Energy Index)

weight	weight fa	food name	calories	sugars	total carl	fiber	protein	energy index	protein index
149	1.49	prickly pear fruit	61	0	14.3	5.4	1.1	-0.373	0.750
130	1.3	beans-black-canned	110	1	19	7	7	-0.354	2.541
100	1	agave hearts	68	3	16	7	1	-0.080	0.465
23	0.23	fireweed-leaves	24	0	4.4	2.4	1.1	0.042	1.600
247	2.47	soup-blackbean	116	0	19.8	4.4	5.6	0.156	1.102
10	0.1	lettuce-romaine	2	0	0.3	0.2	0.1	0.184	0.585
100	1	amaranth-raw	25	0	3.9	0	2.5	0.250	1.549
110	1.1	beans-green-snap	34	1.5	7.9	3.7	2	0.357	0.701
246	2.46	Hummus	435	1.1	49.5	9.8	12	0.386	1.234
245	2.45	milk-soy	120	1.2	11.4	3.2	9.2	0.519	2.044
104	1.04	taro-raw	116	0.4	27.5	4.3	1.6	0.558	-0.136
62	0.62	cauliflower (cooked)	14	0.9	2.5	1.7	1.1	0.620	0.644
58	0.58	potato-baked	77	0	17.2	3.2	2.5	0.621	0.466
251	2.51	soup-clam chowder	176	0	21.8	1.5	10.9	0.665	1.659
120	1.2	celery-raw	17	2.2	3.6	1.9	0.8	0.755	-0.242
100	1	asparagus	20	1.9	3.9	2.1	2.2	0.784	0.799
10	0.1	kelp-raw	4	0.1	1	0.1	0.2	0.796	0.204
100	1	broccoli-raw	35	1.8	6.4	2.6	3	0.800	1.030
55	0.55	lettuce-iceberg	6	1	1.1	0.6	0.4	0.810	-0.204
631	6.31	pizza-whole-cheese,veggies, mea	1470	13	170.1	19	103.9	0.865	3.590
240	2.4	soup-beef with vegetables	170	1.6	19.6	1.4	11.7	0.942	1.741
43	0.43	purslane	43	0	1.5	0	0.6	1.000	0.034
696	6.96	spaghetti with meat sauce	640	17	92	12	23	1.069	0.354
255	2.55	salad-greek with feta	268	2	8.8	3.6	8.9	1.161	1.433
151	1.51	bamboo shoots	41	4.5	7.9	3.3	3.9	1.175	0.521
639	6.39	spaghetti with marinara	490	17	90	10	14	1.205	-0.295
240	2.4	soup-vegetable	122	4.4	19	1.2	3.5	1.218	-0.404
100	1	cereal-cheerios	393	3.3	73.3	10	10	1.250	-0.050
100	1	blackberries	43	4.9	9.6	5.3	1.4	1.266	-0.552
25	0.25	persimmons	32	0	8.4	0	0.2	1.280	-1.097
85	0.85	oatmeal-multigrain prepared	52	1.9	11.5	1.9	1.8	1.336	-0.436
118	1.18	burdock-raw	85	3.4	20.5	3.9	1.8	1.357	-0.800
160	1.6	egg noodles	213	0.5	39.7	1.8	7.6	1.375	-0.011
124	1.24	peas-green-sweet	70	4	11	3	4	1.565	0.145
30	0.3	salsa-tomato	10	1	2	0	0	1.667	-1.667
55	0.55	dandelion greens- raw	25	2.1	5.1	1.9	1.5	1.719	-0.304
128	1.28	carrots	52	5.8	12.3	3.8	1.2	1.768	-1.289
133	1.33	sweet potato-raw	101	5.2	23.4	4	2.1	1.842	-1.270
100	1	bread-wheat	260	0	47	4.3	4	1.860	-1.159
152	1.52	strawberries	49	7.1	11.7	3	1	1.954	-1.582
160	1.6	onion	67	6.8	16.2	2.2	1.5	1.998	-1.532
200	2	chickpeas	728	0	45.2	8.8	10	2.091	-0.557
213	2.13	meatloaf-double sauced with grav	360	3	19	1	23	2.235	3.472
231	2.31	burrito-bean	508	3	66	5	22.5	2.286	0.240
91	0.91	fish fillet-breaded-fried	211	0	15.4	0.5	13.3	2.308	3.121
40	0.4	peanuts-shelled	90	0.7	6	2.5	3.8	2.325	1.475
245	2.45	milk-skim or fatfree	83	12.5	12.2	0	8.3	2.380	-0.118
100	1	bread-french	243	0	54.1	0	1.4	2.430	-2.212
95	0.95	almonds	549	4.6	18.8	11.2	20.2	2.434	4.704
248	2.48	sou-tomato	161	12.2	22.3	2.7	6.1	2.499	-1.204
100	1	bread-pita	275	0	56	2	9	2.590	-1.226
154	1.54	watermelon	46	9.5	11.6	0.6	0.9	2.757	-2.424
245	2.45	salad-fruit	74	16	19.3	2.5	0.9	2.812	-2.607
29	0.29	Triscuit-ruduced fat	120	0	21	3	3	2.897	-1.641
151	1.51	hummus and feta bagel	279	5	45	3	9	2.934	-1.436
200	2	rice-short-grain white	716	0	158.3	5.6	13	2.953	-2.224
402	4.02	Thai Chicken Pizza	663	16	89	5	40	2.993	0.103
28	0.28	Triscuit-romsemary&olive	120	0	20	3	3	3.000	-1.684
100	1	pretzels-large soft	277	1.6	56.3	3.1	9.4	3.026	-1.608
240	2.4	milk-1% milkfat	130	15	16	0	11	3.042	-0.292

LoS Hi-Fi foods (In alphabetical order)

weight	weight fa	food name	calories	sugars	total carl	fiber	protein	energy index	protein index
28.3	0.283	acorns-oak-raw	110	0	11.5	0	1.7	3.887	-2.701
100	1	agave hearts	68	3	16	7	1	-0.080	0.465
95	0.95	almonds	549	4.6	18.8	11.2	20.2	2.434	4.704
100	1	amaranth-raw	25	0	3.9	0	2.5	0.250	1.549
125	1.25	apple	65	13	17.3	3	0.3	4.392	-4.291
100	1	asparagus	20	1.9	3.9	2.1	2.2	0.784	0.799
151	1.51	bamboo shoots	41	4.5	7.9	3.3	3.9	1.175	0.521
130	1.3	beans-black-canned	110	1	19	7	7	-0.354	2.541
110	1.1	beans-green-snap	34	1.5	7.9	3.7	2	0.357	0.701
100	1	blackberries	43	4.9	9.6	5.3	1.4	1.266	-0.552
145	1.45	blueberries	83	14.4	21	3.5	1.1	4.207	-3.897
100	1	bread-french	243	0	54.1	0	1.4	2.430	-2.212
100	1	bread-pita	275	0	56	2	9	2.590	-1.226
100	1	bread-wheat	260	0	47	4.3	4	1.860	-1.159
45	0.45	bread-white	132	2.1	24.5	1.1	4	4.692	-3.313
100	1	broccoli-raw	35	1.8	6.4	2.6	3	0.800	1.030
118	1.18	burdock-raw	85	3.4	20.5	3.9	1.8	1.357	-0.800
231	2.31	burrito-bean	508	3	66	5	22.5	2.286	0.240
177	1.77	cantaloupe	60	13.9	14.4	1.6	1.5	3.422	-2.955
128	1.28	carrots	52	5.8	12.3	3.8	1.2	1.768	-1.289
62	0.62	cauliflower (cooked)	14	0.9	2.5	1.7	1.1	0.620	0.644
120	1.2	celery-raw	17	2.2	3.6	1.9	0.8	0.755	-0.242
100	1	cereal-cheerios	393	3.3	73.3	10	10	1.250	-0.050
232	2.32	cheese-cream	810	6.2	6.2	0	17.5	4.560	1.392
200	2	chickpeas	728	0	45.2	8.8	10	2.091	-0.557
80	0.8	coconut-meat	283	5	12.2	7.2	2.7	3.446	-2.109
240	2.4	coconut-milk	552	8	13.3	5.3	5.5	3.165	-1.691
28.3	0.283	corn nuts	126	0.2	20.3	2	2.4	4.170	-3.132
100	1	crackers-saltines	393	0	82	2.7	10.5	3.638	-2.497
55	0.55	dandelion greens- raw	25	2.1	5.1	1.9	1.5	1.719	-0.304
160	1.6	egg noodles	213	0.5	39.7	1.8	7.6	1.375	-0.011
23	0.23	fireweed-leaves	24	0	4.4	2.4	1.1	0.042	1.600
91	0.91	fish fillet-breaded-fried	211	0	15.4	0.5	13.3	2.308	3.121
115	1.15	hazelnuts	722	5	19.2	11.2	17.2	3.654	1.948
246	2.46	Hummus	435	1.1	49.5	9.8	12	0.386	1.234
151	1.51	hummus and feta bagel	279	5	45	3	9	2.934	-1.436
10	0.1	kelp-raw	4	0.1	1	0.1	0.2	0.796	0.204
55	0.55	lettuce-iceberg	6	1	1.1	0.6	0.4	0.810	-0.204
10	0.1	lettuce-romaine	2	0	0.3	0.2	0.1	0.184	0.585
213	2.13	meatloaf-double sauced with grav	360	3	19	1	23	2.235	3.472
240	2.4	milk-1% milkfat	130	15	16	0	11	3.042	-0.292
245	2.45	milk-skim or fatfree	83	12.5	12.2	0	8.3	2.380	-0.118
245	2.45	milk-soy	120	1.2	11.4	3.2	9.2	0.519	2.044
100	1	mulberries-raw	43	8.1	9.8	1.7	1.4	3.554	-2.847
28.3	0.283	oak-acorns-raw	110	0	11.5	0	1.7	3.887	-2.701
155	1.55	oatmeal-maple and brown sugar	157	12.6	31.1	2.8	3.7	4.062	-3.268
85	0.85	oatmeal-multigrain prepared	52	1.9	11.5	1.9	1.8	1.336	-0.436
160	1.6	onion	67	6.8	16.2	2.2	1.5	1.998	-1.532
185	1.85	orange	85	16.9	21.3	4.4	1.3	3.695	-3.368
258	2.58	peanutbutter-chunky	1520	20.1	54.4	17	64.7	4.527	3.540
40	0.4	peanuts-shelled	90	0.7	6	2.5	3.8	2.325	1.475
124	1.24	peas-green-sweet	70	4	11	3	4	1.565	0.145
25	0.25	persimmons	32	0	8.4	0	0.2	1.280	-1.097
155	1.55	pineapple	74	14.4	19.6	2.2	0.8	4.069	-3.841
128	1.28	pistachio-dry roasted	731	10	35.4	13.2	27.3	3.391	2.273
146	1.46	pizza-slice-pepperoni	400	3	36.2	2.3	16.2	3.417	-0.228
631	6.31	pizza-whole-cheese,veggies, mea	1470	13	170.1	19	103.9	0.865	3.590
8	0.08	popcorn (air popped)	31	0.1	6.2	1.2	1	3.655	-2.226
11	0.11	popcorn (oil popped)	55	0.1	6.3	1.1	1	4.924	-3.572
58	0.58	potato-baked	77	0	17.2	3.2	2.5	0.621	0.466

High Protein Dinner Foods

These foods should be eaten after exercise, preferably in the evening a couple hours before sleep. Most high-protein foods (those with a Protein Index of 10 or higher) should be the main course and can be accompanied by moderately high protein foods (protein index between 2 and 10) and some low protein foods (protein index between 0 and 2). In order to calculate the percentage of your dinner that is protein you can use a simple guide: if all the foods are about the same amount of servings, add up all their protein indexes and add up all the energy indexes combined (if either number is negative, use .1). You should have a protein number and an energy number; add the two figures and divide the protein number by that number. That is your protein percentage.

Let's use a chicken burrito as an example. It's made up of basically three components: chicken, cheese, and the tortilla wrap.

chicken: Protein Index (PI): 27.029, Energy Index (EI): -3.877
cheese: PI: 20.190, EI: 2.667
wrap: PI -2.187, EI: 3.649

Protein = 27.029 + 20.190 - 2.187 = 45.032
Energy = (-3.877) + 2.667 + 2.187 = .977
Total = 46.009
Protein Percentage = 45.032 / 46.009 = 97.9% (That's really high!)

The Evolution Diet uses the Food Guide Pyramid as a guide for serving size. All of these are considered one serving:
1 slice bread
1 ounce of ready to eat cereal
1/2 cup of cooked cereal, rice, or pasta
1 cup of raw, leafy vegetables
1/2 cup other vegetables, cooked or chopped

1 medium apple, banana, orange
3/4 cup fruit juice
1 cup milk
2 oz cheese
2-3 oz of cooked lean meat, poultry, or fish
1/2 cup cooked dry beans or 1 egg counts as 1 oz of lean meat
2 tablespoons of peanut butter or 1/3 cup of nuts count as 1 oz
of lean meat.

Some High Protein Foods also have a high energy index (e.g. beef jerky or peanut butter) and should be eaten sparingly to avoid contradictory digestive reactions.

High protein foods are generally high in nutrition as well as protein. The fish that make up most of the top protein foods are high in essential fatty acids and essential amino acids. These foods are vital to our existence and should be eaten regularly.

The charts that follow are the high protein foods listed, first, in order of protein index and second, in alphabetical order.

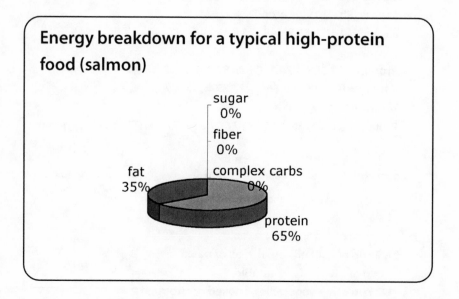

Energy breakdown for a typical high-protein food (salmon)

sugar 0%
fiber 0%
complex carbs 0%
fat 35%
protein 65%

High-protein foods (In order by Protein Index)

weight	weight fa	food name	calories	sugars	total carl	fiber	protein	energy index	protein index
85	0.85	fish-tuna-bluefin	156	0	0	0	25.4	1.835	28.047
140	1.4	chicken-meat only-roasted	266	0	0	0	40.5	1.900	27.029
56	0.56	tuna-canned-in water	70	0	0	0	15	1.250	25.536
155	1.55	fish-salmon wild coho	285	0	0	0	42.4	1.839	25.516
85	0.85	pork loin	203	0	0	0	23.1	2.388	24.788
106	1.06	fish-swordfish-cooked	164	0	0	0	26.9	1.547	23.830
283	2.83	beef-select-cooked	824	0	0	0	74.1	2.912	23.272
154	1.54	fish-whitefish	265	0	0	0	37.7	1.721	22.760
101	1.01	fish-sea bass	125	0	0	0	23.9	1.238	22.426
180	1.8	fish-cod-atlantic-cooked	189	0	0	0	41.1	1.050	21.783
30	0.3	cheese-mozarella	80	0	0.5	0	8	2.667	20.190
178	1.78	fish-salmon-atlantic-cooked	367	0	0	0	39.3	2.062	20.017
85	0.85	shrimp	84	0	0	0	17.8	0.988	19.953
269	2.69	beef-ribs-broiled	920	0	0	0	59.8	3.420	18.810
136	1.36	sushi-swordfish	165	0	0	0	26.9	1.213	18.566
134	1.34	crab	130	0	0	0	25.9	0.970	18.358
198	1.98	sushi-salmon	362	0	0	0	39.4	1.828	18.071
85	0.85	fish-orange roughy	76	0	0	0	16	0.894	17.929
28.3	0.283	sushi-flounder	26	0	0	0	5.3	0.919	17.809
32	0.32	chicken wings- no sauce	103	0	0.8	0	8.4	3.219	17.781
136	1.36	fish-salmon-smoked	159	0	0	0	24.9	1.169	17.140
145	1.45	lobster	142	0	1.9	0	29.7	0.979	17.130
240	2.4	cheese-brie	802	1.1	1.1	0	49.8	3.525	16.316
320	3.2	beef-corned	803	0	1.5	0	58.1	2.509	14.834
151	1.51	fish-sablefish	378	0	0	0	26	2.503	14.715
85	0.85	mussel-blue	146	0	6.3	0.2	20.2	1.716	11.933
84	0.84	chicken-fried breast with skin	218	0	7.6	0.3	20.9	2.591	10.472
243	2.43	eggs	357	1.9	1.9	0	30.6	1.782	9.897
126	1.26	tofu-raw	183	0	5.4	2.9	19.9	1.185	9.870
100	1	eggs-hard-boiled	155	0	1.1	0	12.5	1.550	9.711
243	2.43	egg-white-fresh	126	1.7	1.8	0	26.5	0.798	9.355
113	1.13	chicken-meat and skin-fried	313	0	10.7	0	26.6	2.770	9.321
226	2.26	cheese-cottage	203	0.7	8.2	0	31.1	1.022	9.075
226	2.26	cottage cheese	203	0.7	8.2	0	31.1	1.022	9.075
28.3	0.283	beef jerky	116	2.5	3.1	0.5	9.4	7.597	8.254
243	2.43	egg-yolk-fresh	782	1.4	8.7	0	38.5	3.449	8.218
15	0.15	eggs-omelet-just egg	23	0.1	0.1	0	1.6	1.800	8.200
87	0.87	fish-catfish-breaded-fried	199	0	7	0.6	15.7	2.271	7.729
73	0.73	chicken wings-with babrbeque sa	160	3	5	0	14	3.836	7.546
61	0.61	eggs-egg beaters	30	1	1	0	6	1.148	7.303
256	2.56	beans-soy-raw	376	0	28.3	10.8	33.2	-0.354	6.513
172	1.72	beans-black-cooked	227	1	40.8	15	15.2	-3.680	6.301
205	2.05	tuna salad	383	1	19.3	2	32.9	1.985	6.281
150	1.5	cheese-feta	396	6.1	6.1	0	21.3	4.267	5.828
263	2.63	chili-beef and vegetable	339	2.9	42.9	19.2	13.4	-3.877	5.813
180	1.8	edemame (soybeans)	254	0	19.9	7.6	22.2	0.128	5.730
226	2.26	cottage cheese with fruit	219	5.4	10.4	0.5	24.2	1.920	5.413
259	2.59	hamburger-tripple patty with top|	692	7	34.2	3	50	3.614	4.706

High-protein foods (In order by Protein Index)

weight	weight fa	food name	calories	sugars	total carl	fiber	protein	energy index	protein index
172	1.72	beans-black-cooked	227	1	40.8	15	15.2	-3.680	6.301
256	2.56	beans-soy-raw	376	0	28.3	10.8	33.2	-0.354	6.513
28.3	0.283	beef jerky	116	2.5	3.1	0.5	9.4	7.597	8.254
320	3.2	beef-corned	803	0	1.5	0	58.1	2.509	14.834
269	2.69	beef-ribs-broiled	920	0	0	0	59.8	3.420	18.810
283	2.83	beef-select-cooked	824	0	0	0	74.1	2.912	23.272
240	2.4	cheese-brie	802	1.1	1.1	0	49.8	3.525	16.316
226	2.26	cheese-cottage	203	0.7	8.2	0	31.1	1.022	9.075
150	1.5	cheese-feta	396	6.1	6.1	0	21.3	4.267	5.828
30	0.3	cheese-mozarella	80	0	0.5	0	8	2.667	20.190
32	0.32	chicken wings- no sauce	103	0	0.8	0	8.4	3.219	17.781
73	0.73	chicken wings-with babrbeque sa	160	3	5	0	14	3.836	7.546
84	0.84	chicken-fried breast with skin	218	0	7.6	0.3	20.9	2.591	10.472
113	1.13	chicken-meat and skin-fried	313	0	10.7	0	26.6	2.770	9.321
140	1.4	chicken-meat only-roasted	266	0	0	0	40.5	1.900	27.029
263	2.63	chili-beef and vegetable	339	2.9	42.9	19.2	13.4	-3.877	5.813
226	2.26	cottage cheese	203	0.7	8.2	0	31.1	1.022	9.075
226	2.26	cottage cheese with fruit	219	5.4	10.4	0.5	24.2	1.920	5.413
134	1.34	crab	130	0	0	0	25.9	0.970	18.358
180	1.8	edamame (soybeans)	254	0	19.9	7.6	22.2	0.128	5.730
243	2.43	eggs	357	1.9	1.9	0	30.6	1.782	9.897
61	0.61	eggs-egg beaters	30	1	1	0	6	1.148	7.303
100	1	eggs-hard-boiled	155	0	1.1	0	12.5	1.550	9.711
15	0.15	eggs-omelet-just egg	23	0.1	0.1	0	1.6	1.800	8.200
243	2.43	egg-white-fresh	126	1.7	1.8	0	26.5	0.798	9.355
243	2.43	egg-yolk-fresh	782	1.4	8.7	0	38.5	3.449	8.218
87	0.87	fish-catfish-breaded-fried	199	0	7	0.6	15.7	2.271	7.729
180	1.8	fish-cod-atlantic-cooked	189	0	0	0	41.1	1.050	21.783
85	0.85	fish-orange roughy	76	0	0	0	16	0.894	17.929
151	1.51	fish-sablefish	378	0	0	0	26	2.503	14.715
155	1.55	fish-salmon wild coho	285	0	0	0	42.4	1.839	25.516
178	1.78	fish-salmon-atlantic-cooked	367	0	0	0	39.3	2.062	20.017
136	1.36	fish-salmon-smoked	159	0	0	0	24.9	1.169	17.140
101	1.01	fish-sea bass	125	0	0	0	23.9	1.238	22.426
106	1.06	fish-swordfish-cooked	164	0	0	0	26.9	1.547	23.830
85	0.85	fish-tuna-bluefin	156	0	0	0	25.4	1.835	28.047
154	1.54	fish-whitefish	265	0	0	0	37.7	1.721	22.760
259	2.59	hamburger-tripple patty with topj	692	7	34.2	3	50	3.614	4.706
145	1.45	lobster	142	0	1.9	0	29.7	0.979	17.130
85	0.85	mussel-blue	146	0	6.3	0.2	20.2	1.716	11.933
85	0.85	pork loin	203	0	0	0	23.1	2.388	24.788
85	0.85	shrimp	84	0	0	0	17.8	0.988	19.953
28.3	0.283	sushi-flounder	26	0	0	0	5.3	0.919	17.809
198	1.98	sushi-salmon	362	0	0	0	39.4	1.828	18.071
136	1.36	sushi-swordfish	165	0	0	0	26.9	1.213	18.566
126	1.26	tofu-raw	183	0	5.4	2.9	19.9	1.185	9.870
205	2.05	tuna salad	383	1	19.3	2	32.9	1.985	6.281
56	0.56	tuna-canned-in water	70	0	0	0	15	1.250	25.536

High Energy Foods

When you are about to exercise (and you don't want to lose weight), you may want a little boost so that your muscles will perform at the top of their ability. High Energy Foods are full of instant energy because they are loaded with simple sugars.

It doesn't take long for your body to realize the affects of these foods, so you should eat them only when you need an immediate boost. This may happen when you're a little sluggish or tired. A small glass of orange juice may be just what the doctor ordered in the morning to accompany your LoS Hi-Fi breakfast, but a large bowl of extremely sugary cereal is not called for. When you take in too much of these foods, you will overload your system and most of it will go straight to fat.

Additionally, eating these foods at the wrong time can cause irritability, anxiousness, and soon after energy lulls and fatigue. Becoming dependent on these food also has its adverse effects. These are the foods that, when eaten often in mass quantities, result in diabetes and other diseases.

Eat these in extreme moderation before or during physical activity.

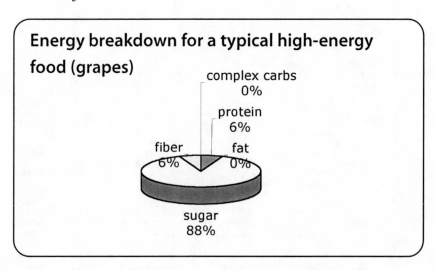

Energy breakdown for a typical high-energy food (grapes)

complex carbs 0%
protein 6%
fiber 6%
fat 0%
sugar 88%

High-energy foods (In order by Energy Index)

weight	weight fa	food name	calories	sugars	total carl	fiber	protein	energy index	protein index
178	1.78	dates	502	112.8	133.6	14.2	4.4	23.637	-23.347
57	0.57	popcorn with caramel topping	228	27.2	46	2.2	3.6	22.748	-22.052
277	2.77	cranberry sauce	418	105	107.8	2.8	0.6	16.558	-16.514
60	0.6	granola	220	17	48	3	4.8	14.400	-13.511
28.3	0.283	cookies-oatmeal	127	7	19.4	0.8	1.8	14.291	-13.481
28	0.28	grahams crackers (Nabisco)	119	6.4	21.3	1	2	13.250	-12.420
100	1	v-8 Splash	110	27	27	0	0	11.900	-11.900
146	1.46	trail mix	707	27	65.6	7	20.7	10.897	-8.316
30	0.3	cereal-multigrain cheerios	110	6	24	3	3	10.467	-9.356
100	1	cereal-raisin bran	317	33	79	13	8	9.610	-8.711
100	1	orange juice	105	20.9	24.5	0.5	1.5	9.400	-8.965
32	0.32	peanutbutter-creamy	190	3	7	2	8	9.188	-1.344
30	0.3	cereal-Wheaties	107	4.2	24.3	3	3	7.967	-6.868
28.3	0.283	cashew-raw (steamed)	160	1.7	7.7	0.9	5.2	7.942	-3.004
30	0.3	wasabi peas	80	4	12	1	1	7.867	-7.200
30	0.3	crackers-TLC-original 7 grain	130	3	22	2	3	7.800	-6.600
70	0.7	macaroni and cheese-kraft	260	7	48	1	9	7.657	-6.021
28.3	0.283	beef jerky	116	2.5	3.1	0.5	9.4	7.597	8.254
129	1.29	cashews-oil roasted	749	6.5	38.9	4.3	21.7	7.248	-3.059
92	0.92	grapes	62	14.9	15.8	0.8	0.6	7.124	-6.884
100	1	sugarcane	64	16	16	0	0	7.040	-7.040
65	0.65	corn bread	173	8	28.3	3	4.4	7.031	-5.766
694	6.94	smoothie made with yogurt	480	102	110	4	10	6.478	-5.921
228	2.28	sweet potato-candied	203	35.1	47.7	5.7	2.2	6.478	-6.166
165	1.65	mango	107	24.4	28.1	3	0.8	6.345	-6.166
28	0.28	cereal- Kellogg's Corn Flakes	101	2	24.1	1	2	6.321	-5.578
28	0.28	peanuts-salted	170	0.5	6	2	7	6.214	1.740
28.3	0.283	Chex mix	120	1.6	18.4	1.6	3.1	6.140	-4.680
248	2.48	lemonade	131	32.6	34.1	0.2	0.2	5.786	-5.752
28.3	0.283	beechnut- dried	163	0	9.5	1.3	1.8	5.521	-4.061
120	1.2	walnuts	785	3.1	16.5	8	18.3	5.442	0.979
225	2.25	banana	200	27.5	51.4	5.8	2.5	5.180	-4.841
248	2.48	apple juice	117	28.8	29	0.2	0.1	5.116	-5.098

High-energy foods (In alphabetical order)

weight	weight fa	food name	calories	sugars	total carl	fiber	protein	energy index	protein index
248	2.48	apple juice	117	28.8	29	0.2	0.1	5.116	-5.098
225	2.25	banana	200	27.5	51.4	5.8	2.5	5.180	-4.841
28.3	0.283	beechnut- dried	163	0	9.5	1.3	1.8	5.521	-4.061
28.3	0.283	beef jerky	116	2.5	3.1	0.5	9.4	7.597	8.254
28.3	0.283	cashew-raw (steamed)	160	1.7	7.7	0.9	5.2	7.942	-3.004
129	1.29	cashews-oil roasted	749	6.5	38.9	4.3	21.7	7.248	-3.059
28	0.28	cereal- Kellogg's Corn Flakes	101	2	24.1	1	2	6.321	-5.578
30	0.3	cereal-multigrain cheerios	110	6	24	3	3	10.467	-9.356
100	1	cereal-raisin bran	317	33	79	13	8	9.610	-8.711
30	0.3	cereal-Wheaties	107	4.2	24.3	3	3	7.967	-6.868
28.3	0.283	Chex mix	120	1.6	18.4	1.6	3.1	6.140	-4.680
28.3	0.283	cookies-oatmeal	127	7	19.4	0.8	1.8	14.291	-13.481
65	0.65	corn bread	173	8	28.3	3	4.4	7.031	-5.766
30	0.3	crackers-TLC-original 7 grain	130	3	22	2	3	7.800	-6.600
277	2.77	cranberry sauce	418	105	107.8	2.8	0.6	16.558	-16.514
178	1.78	dates	502	112.8	133.6	14.2	4.4	23.637	-23.347
28	0.28	grahams crackers (Nabisco)	119	6.4	21.3	1	2	13.250	-12.420
60	0.6	granola	220	17	48	3	4.8	14.400	-13.511
92	0.92	grapes	62	14.9	15.8	0.8	0.6	7.124	-6.884
248	2.48	lemonade	131	32.6	34.1	0.2	0.2	5.786	-5.752
70	0.7	macaroni and cheese-kraft	260	7	48	1	9	7.657	-6.021
165	1.65	mango	107	24.4	28.1	3	0.8	6.345	-6.166
100	1	orange juice	105	20.9	24.5	0.5	1.5	9.400	-8.965
32	0.32	peanutbutter-creamy	190	3	7	2	8	9.188	-1.344
28	0.28	peanuts-salted	170	0.5	6	2	7	6.214	1.740
57	0.57	popcorn with caramel topping	228	27.2	46	2.2	3.6	22.748	-22.052
694	6.94	smoothie made with yogurt	480	102	110	4	10	6.478	-5.921
100	1	sugarcane	64	16	16	0	0	7.040	-7.040
228	2.28	sweet potato-candied	203	35.1	47.7	5.7	2.2	6.478	-6.166
146	1.46	trail mix	707	27	65.6	7	20.7	10.897	-8.316
100	1	v-8 Splash	110	27	27	0	0	11.900	-11.900
120	1.2	walnuts	785	3.1	16.5	8	18.3	5.442	0.979
30	0.3	wasabi peas	80	4	12	1	1	7.867	-7.200

Foods to be avoided (In order by Energy Index)

weight	weight fa	food name	calories	sugars	total carl	fiber	protein	energy index	protein index
100	1	Snickers bar	477	51.1	59.6	1.7	6.8	25.094	-24.117
30	0.3	cereal-Frosted Wheaties	112	11.7	26.7	0.6	1.2	19.285	-18.881
27	0.27	cereal-peanutbutter crunch	120	10	22	1	2	19.111	-18.301
100	1	cereal-cinnamon toast crunch	440	34	79	4	5	17.360	-16.798
100	1	Pop Tart	404	30.8	71.2	1	3.8	16.320	-15.852
100	1	Chocolate Oreo Mudslide Cheesec	389	28.5	36.7	1.5	5.2	15.200	-14.087
28.3	0.283	danish pastry	105	7.8	13.5	0.5	1.5	14.700	-13.781
28.3	0.283	doughnut	119	6.4	14.1	0.4	1.4	13.228	-12.401
100	1	Starbuck's blueberry muffin	303	20.4	45.8	1.4	4.9	11.112	-10.233
100	1	yogurt-low fat	102	19.1	19.1	0	4.4	8.660	-7.148
100	1	Red Bull	64	15.6	16	0	0.2	6.880	-6.803
100	1	Doritos	493	3.5	59.9	3.5	7	5.840	-4.839
250	2.5	smoothie café mocha	225	30.8	34	0	7.8	5.828	-4.506
100	1	Starbuck's caramel Frappuccino	71	11	12.8	0	2.1	5.110	-4.189
100	1	cola	40	11.3	11.3	0	0	4.920	-4.920
100	1	Lay's potato chips	536	0	53.6	3.6	7.1	4.842	-3.725
314	3.14	Burger King's Whopper	760	11	52	3	33	3.707	0.250
185	1.85	fish-battered fillet sandwich	520	4	44	2	18	3.589	-0.709
98	0.98	hotdog-plain	242	3	18	2	10.4	3.531	0.210
100	1	chicken nuggets	308	0	17.6	0	15.4	3.080	2.500
170	1.7	McDonald's French fries- large	570	0	70	7	6	2.200	-1.510

Foods to be avoided (In alphabetical order)

weight	weight fa	food name	calories	sugars	total carl	fiber	protein	energy index	protein index
314	3.14	Burger King's Whopper	760	11	52	3	33	3.707	0.250
100	1	cereal-cinnamon toast crunch	440	34	79	4	5	17.360	-16.798
30	0.3	cereal-Frosted Wheaties	112	11.7	26.7	0.6	1.2	19.285	-18.881
27	0.27	cereal-peanutbutter crunch	120	10	22	1	2	19.111	-18.301
100	1	chicken nuggets	308	0	17.6	0	15.4	3.080	2.500
100	1	Chocolate Oreo Mudslide Cheesec	389	28.5	36.7	1.5	5.2	15.200	-14.087
100	1	cola	40	11.3	11.3	0	0	4.920	-4.920
28.3	0.283	danish pastry	105	7.8	13.5	0.5	1.5	14.700	-13.781
100	1	Doritos	493	3.5	59.9	3.5	7	5.840	-4.839
28.3	0.283	doughnut	119	6.4	14.1	0.4	1.4	13.228	-12.401
185	1.85	fish-battered fillet sandwich	520	4	44	2	18	3.589	-0.709
98	0.98	hotdog-plain	242	3	18	2	10.4	3.531	0.210
100	1	Lay's potato chips	536	0	53.6	3.6	7.1	4.842	-3.725
170	1.7	McDonald's French fries- large	570	0	70	7	6	2.200	-1.510
100	1	Pop Tart	404	30.8	71.2	1	3.8	16.320	-15.852
100	1	Red Bull	64	15.6	16	0	0.2	6.880	-6.803
250	2.5	smoothie café mocha	225	30.8	34	0	7.8	5.828	-4.506
100	1	Snickers bar	477	51.1	59.6	1.7	6.8	25.094	-24.117
100	1	Starbuck's blueberry muffin	303	20.4	45.8	1.4	4.9	11.112	-10.233
100	1	Starbuck's caramel Frappuccino	71	11	12.8	0	2.1	5.110	-4.189
100	1	yogurt-low fat	102	19.1	19.1	0	4.4	8.660	-7.148

Calorie Expenditures for Various Physical Activites (1 Hour)

BODY WEIGHT LB	97	110	123	137	159	163	176	190	203	216	229	242	255	269
Badminton	265	300	325	360	395	430	465	500	535	570	600	635	665	700
Baseball	210	225	240	255	270	285	290	305	320	335	350	365	380	395
Basketball	365	415	460	510	565	610	660	710	760	805	855	905	950	995
Competitive	390	445	500	550	600	655	710	760	810	865	910	960	1010	1065
Boxing	400	455	510	565	620	675	730	785	840	895	950	1005	1055	1110
Circuit Training	350	380	410	440	470	500	530	560	590	620	650	680	710	740
Cycle @ 12 mph	360	390	425	460	495	530	565	600	635	670	705	740	775	810
Racing	450	510	570	630	690	750	810	870	930	990	1050	1110	1170	1230
Dancing	270	295	320	345	370	395	420	445	470	495	520	545	570	595
Golf	230	260	290	320	350	380	410	440	470	500	530	560	590	620
Horse Riding	240	275	310	345	370	405	440	475	510	545	580	615	650	685

BODY WEIGHT LB	97	110	123	137	159	163	176	190	203	216	229	242	255	269
Rowing Crew	600	660	720	780	830	890	940	1000	1060	1120	1180	1235	1295	1345
Running @ 6.5 mph	425	480	535	590	650	705	760	820	875	930	985	1045	1100	1160
@ 10 mph	620	690	765	835	900	965	1035	1100	1170	1235	1300	1365	1430	1495
Skating (inline)	250	285	320	355	380	410	445	480	515	550	590	625	660	700
Skiing (piste)	295	335	375	415	455	495	535	575	615	655	695	735	775	815
Soccer	355	400	445	490	535	580	625	670	715	760	805	850	895	940
Squash	515	580	645	710	785	850	915	980	1045	1110	1175	1240	1305	1370
Swimming Slow	230	260	290	320	350	380	410	440	470	500	530	560	590	620
Fast laps	400	445	490	535	580	625	670	705	750	795	840	885	930	975
Tennis social	300	340	375	415	455	490	530	570	605	645	680	720	760	795
Weight Training	350	395	440	485	530	575	620	665	710	755	800	845	890	935
Walking 5 kph.	200	220	240	260	280	300	320	340	360	380	400	420	440	460

Note: Figures are just estimates and may not be completely accurate. Muscle mass and activity level play a part in determining the acctual calorie expenditure.

Universal Edibility Test

1 Test only one part of a potential food plant at a time.

2 Separate the plant into its basic components - leaves, stems, roots, buds, and flowers.

3 Smell the food for strong or acid odors. Remember, smell alone does not indicate a plant is edible or inedible.

4 Do not eat for 8 hours before starting the test.

5 During the 8 hours you abstain from eating, test for contact poisoning by placing a piece of the plant part you are testing on the inside of your elbow or wrist. Usually 15 minutes is enough time to allow for a reaction.

6 During the test period, take nothing by mouth except purified water and the plant part you are testing.

7 Select a small portion of a single part and prepare it the way you plan to eat it.

8 Before placing the prepared plant part in your mouth, touch a small portion (a pinch) to the outer surface of your lip to test for burning or itching.

9 If after 3 minutes there is no reaction on your lip, place the plant part on your tongue, holding it there for 15 minutes.

10 If there is no reaction, thoroughly chew a pinch and hold it in your mouth for 15 minutes. Do not swallow.

11 If no burning, itching, numbing, stinging, or other irritation occurs during the 15 minutes, swallow the food.

12 Wait 8 hours. If any ill effects occur during this period, induce vomiting and drink a lot of water.

13 If no ill effects occur, eat 0.25 cup of the same plant part prepared the same way. Wait another 8 hours. If no ill effects occur, the plant part as prepared is safe for eating.

Food Allergy Self-Diagnosis

The best method for diagnosing food allergy is to be assessed by an allergist. The allergist will review the patient's history and the symptoms or reactions that have been noted after food ingestion. If the allergist feels the symptoms or reactions are consistent with food allergy, he/she will perform allergy tests.

Examples of allergy testing include:

• Skin prick testing is easy to do and results are available in minutes. Different allergists may use different devices for skin prick testing. Some use a "bifurcated needle", which looks like a fork with 2 prongs. Others use a "multi-test", which may look like a small board with several pins sticking out of it. In these tests, a tiny amount of the suspected allergen is put onto the skin or into a testing device, and the device is placed on the skin to prick, or break through, the top layer of skin. This puts a small amount of the allergen under the skin. A hive will form at any spot where the person is allergic. This test generally yields a positive or negative result. It is good for quickly learning if a person is allergic to a particular food or not, because it detects allergic antibodies known as IgE. Skin tests cannot predict if a reaction would occur or what kind of reaction might occur if a person ingests that particular allergen. They can however confirm an allergy in light of a patient's history of reactions to a particular food. Non-IgE mediated allergies cannot be detected by this method.

• Blood tests are another useful diagnostic tool for evaluating IgE-mediated food allergies. For example, the RAST (RadioAllergo-Sorbent Test) detects the presence of IgE antibodies to a particular allergen. A CAP-RAST test is a specific type of RAST test with greater specificity: it can show the amount of IgE present to each allergen. Researchers have been able to determine "predictive values" for certain foods. These predictive values can be compared to the RAST blood test results. If a persons RAST score is higher than the predictive value for that food, then there is over a 95 percent chance the person will have an allergic reaction (limited to rash and anaphylaxis reactions) if they ingest that food. Currently, predictive values are available for the following foods: milk, egg, peanut, fish, soy, and wheat. Blood tests allow for hundreds of allergens to be screened from a single sample, and cover food allergies as well as inhalants. However, non-IgE mediated allergies cannot be detected by this method.

• Food challenges, especially double-blind placebo-controlled food challenges (DBPCFC), are the gold standard for diagnosis of food allergies, including most non-IgE mediated reactions. Blind food challenges involve packaging the suspected allergen into a capsule, giving it to the patient, and observing the patient for signs or symptoms of an allergic reaction. Due to the risk of anaphylaxis, food challenges are usually conducted in a hospital environment in the presence of a doctor.

• Additional diagnostic tools for evaluation of eosinophilic or non-IgE mediated reactions include endoscopy, colonoscopy, and biopsy.

Important differential diagnoses are:

• Lactose intolerance; this generally develops later in life but can present in young patients in severe cases. This is due to an enzyme deficiency (lactase) and not allergy. It occurs in many non-Western people.
• Celiac disease; this is an autoimmune disorder triggered by gluten proteins such as gliadin (present in wheat, rye and barley). It is a non-IgE mediated food allergy by definition.
• Irritable bowel syndrome (IBS)
• C1 esterase inhibitor deficiency (hereditary angioedema); this rare disease generally causes attacks of angioedema, but can present solely with abdominal pain and occasional diarrhea.

Elimination Diet

An elimination diet is a method of identifying foods that an individual cannot consume without adverse effects. Adverse effects may be due to food allergy, food intolerance, other physiological mechanisms (such as metabolic or toxins), or a combination of these. When the mechanism is unknown, but a food is suspected, the mechanism may be described as a food sensitivity or a food hypersensitivity. Elimination diets typically involve entirely removing a suspected food from the diet for a period of time from two weeks to two months, and seeing whether symptoms resolve during that time. In extreme cases, an oligoantigenic diet may be tested.

Common reasons for undertaking an elimination diet include suspected food allergies and suspected food intolerances. An elimination diet might remove one or more common foods, such as eggs or milk, or it might remove one or more minor or non-nutritive substances, such as artificial food colorings.

An elimination diet relies on trial and error to identify specific allergies and intolerances. Typically, if symptoms resolve after the removal of a food from the diet, then the food is reintroduced to see whether the symptoms reappear. This challenge-dechallenge-rechallenge approach is particularly useful in cases with intermittent or vague symptoms.

The terms exclusion diet and elimination diet are often used interchangeably in the literature, and there is no standardised terminology. The exclusion diet can be a diagnostic tool or method used temporarily to determine whether a patient's symptoms are food-related. The term elimination diet is also used to describe a "treatment diet", which eliminates certain foods for a patient.

Adverse reactions to food can be due to several mechanisms. Correct identification of the type of reaction in an individual is important, as different approaches to management are required. The area of adverse reactions to food has been controversial and the subject of ongoing research. It has been characterized in the past by lack of universal acceptance of definitions, diagnosis and treatment.

The elimination diet must be comprehensive containing only those foods unlikely to provoke a reaction, but be able to provide complete nutrition and energy, for the weeks it will be applied, professional nutritional advice is needed. Thorough education about the elimination diet is essential to ensure patients and the parents of children with suspected food intolerance understand the importance of complete adherence to the diet. As inadvertent consumption of an offending chemical can prevent resolution of symptoms and render challenge results useless. Whilst on the elimination diet records are kept of all foods eaten, medications taken and severity of any symptoms. Patients are advised that withdrawal symptoms can occur in the first weeks on the elimination diet, some of the patients symptoms can flare or worsen initially before settling. Whilst on the diet some patients become sensitive to fumes and odors, which may cause symptoms. They are advised to avoid such exposures as this can complicate the elimination and challenge procedures. Particularly to petroleum products, paints, cleaning agents, perfumes, smoke and pressure pack sprays. Once the procedure is complete this sensitivity becomes less of a problem.

Clinical improvement usually occurs over a 2 to 4 week period, if there is no change after a strict adherence to the elimination diet and precipitating factors, then food intolerance is unlikely to be the cause. A normal diet can then be resumed by gradually introducing suspected and eliminated foods or chemical group of foods one at a time. Gradually increasing the amount up to high doses over 3 to 7 days to see if exacerbated reactions are provoked before permanently reintroducing that food to the diet. A strict elimination diet is not usually recommended during pregnancy, although a reduction in suspected foods that reduce symptoms can be helpful.

Glossary

adinosine triphosphate
the molecule needed to produce chemical reactions during exercise.

apnea
condition in which the sufferer stops breathing for 10 seconds or longer, 5 to 50 times an hour. Apnea is often experienced during sleep and can be caused by obesity, alcohol, and enlarged nasal tissue among other causes. Effects of apnea can include poor sleep, hypertension, and

appropriate
apply to a specific purpose; with regard to diet—eat certain foods for specific physical activities.

Artificially Extreme Food (AEF)
any man-made food that is highly concentrated (usually involving sugars), and thus, unnatural in its effects on the human body. AEFs are often found in heavily processed foods and at fast food restaurants, but can also be extremely concentrated natural foods. They include

ATP
adinosine triphosphate.

Australopithecus afarensis
ancestral to genus Homo and modern humans. It is believed that A. afarensis was one of the first

basal metabolism
the basic processes of maintaining life like breathing, maintaining body temperature, pumping blood, etc.

basal metabolic rate (BMR)
the rate at which your body burns calories doing basic life-sustaining activities.

Building Materials
amino acids that cells need in order to operate. These building materials can be found mostly in proteins and should eaten after exercise.

calorie
the unit of energy that is contained in any substance. Calories usually refer to 1000 calories and are actually kilocalories. A can of cola with 200 calories actually has 200,000 calories or 200 kilocalories. For the purposes of this book, we refer to kilocalories as calories.

carbohydrate   a structural component of living cells and a source of energy for animals. Simple sugars like table sugar and corn syrup, and complex carbohydrates like starch are all

carnivore   strictly a meat eater.

cholesterol   a type of fat that animals make (humans included) in their liver. Low-density lipoprotein cholesterol (LDL) is the bad cholesterol and is one of the main causes of heart disease in Western culture. Below 130 mg/dL is optimal for most people. High-density lipoprotein (HDL) is the good guy because high levels of it in the bloodstream seem to prevent heart disease. Above 40 mg/dL is optimal.

Cultureless Human   a theoretical human who has no cultural ties instructing him how to live and how to eat. People today cannot be removed from culture, but the culture-less human is a tool that shows how we are designed to eat.

dietary fiber   any complex carbohydrate that human bodies cannot digest. Cellulose is a common form of fiber and is usually found in leafy vegetables. Natural Man's diet was full of dietary fiber, but modern diets are generally deficient in

digestive tract   the area in an animal's body that alters food into something that can be used by the body's cells.

Energy   the substance needed to complete basic life functions. Energy is contained in everything, but humans get our energy from the food we eat. Energy is measured in

essential amino acid   any amino acid that the body cannot produce on its own and is needed in basic life functions.

essential fatty acid   a fatty acid that is required by the body to operate

The Evolution Diet   the plan of eating in a manner human bodies were designed to eat. This involves eating many small portions of low-sugar, high-fiber foods throughout the day and before exercise and a large high-protein meal after

The Evolution Plan   see The Evolution Diet

exercise   physical activity for the benefit of one's body. Culture-less humans exercised by hunting and gathering among other means.

fat   a soft greasy substance found in animal tissue and consisting of a mixture of lipids (mostly triglycerides). Fat contains 9 kilocalories per gram and is easier to digest than protein, but more difficult than carbohydrates. Fat can be found in 4 forms: saturated (solid at room temperature and found mainly in animal products, butter), monounsaturated (liquid at room temperature and found in olive oil), polyunsaturated (liquid at room temperature and found in vegetable oils), cholesterol

fatty acid   any of a class of aliphatic monocarboxylic acids that are part of a lipid molecule. Fatty acids the free fat molecules that are found in the bloodstream. Some fatty acids are essential to good health because they aid in the digestion

frugivore   an animal that usually eats fruit and sometimes eats other plants or small animals.

ghrelin   peptide hormone that has a significant impact on one's appetite by increasing hunger when heavily present in the

glycemic index   a highly criticized gauge of the energy potential of a particular food. The Glycemic index shows how much a particular food will increase a person's blood sugar level.

glycemic load   the rate at which a particular food affects one's blood sugar with regard to its density.

HCl hydrochloric acid. This acid is present in the stomach and breaks down the food we eat. The presence of HCl in the stomach can be altered based on what foods we eat- the more protein we eat, the higher the amount of acid is released. The more acid in the stomach, the lower the pH level. pH=1 is extremely acidic, while pH=14 is extremely

herbivore strictly a plant eater.

hunter/gatherer society social structure for humans before agriculturization. Clans of people would roam for location to location eating the available plantlife (gathering), and hunting nearby animals. This style of living was the norm for humans for 100,000 years before civilizations began. Humans evolved to fit this lifestyle perfectly and are still designed to live

hyperglycemia abnormally high blood sugar usually associated with

hypertension a common disorder in which blood pressure remains abnormally high (a reading of 140/90 mm Hg or greater).

hypoglycemia abnormally low blood sugar usually resulting from excessive insulin or a poor diet. The Evolution Diet prevents this by encouraging a balanced level of energy

kilocalorie 1000 calories.

leptin hormone that is increased with the increased presence of fat and tells the brain that the person is full.

Life Process vitamins and minerals needed for a perfectly healthy life.

LoS Hi-Fi Foods low sugar hi fiber foods, generally consisting of complex carbohydrates with minimal amounts of protein and fats. These foods should be eaten often in low amounts throughout the day, after a small breakfast and before a large high-protein dinner.

low-carb diet
any method of eating that limits the intake of carbohydrates to unnatural proportions. These diets are used, mainly, to take weight off, but also reduce energy and increase the amount of toxins within the body. Some have said this style of eating, "bores us to weight loss."

Natural Man
human kind that does not rely on processed foods. This is a theoretical tool used to illustrate exactly how we should be eating.

omnivore
an animal that eats both meat and plant foods.

oral cavity
the area in an animal's digestive system where the food enters. Carnivores have sharp teeth, herbivores generally have flat teeth.

partially hydrogenated oils
see trans fat.

protein
any of the nitrogenous organic compounds that are vital for living cells. Proteins contain amino acids, some essential for life. Energy can also be derived from protein when needed through protein metabolism. Protein can be found in meats, dairy, eggs, fish, and some vegetables.

serotonin
a neurotransmitter that has a calming effect on humans and naturally lowers brain activity.

sleep apnea
transient cessation of respiration during sleep. This is usually caused by obesity, alcohol use, some pharmaceuticals, or poor diet. The result is poor sleep, high blood toxicity, and lower BMR, among other

trans fat
common name for an unsaturated fat with trans-isomer fatty acids. Trans fats are generally created by partially hydrogenating plant oils, a process which makes the fat more unhealthy by increasing the chance of coronary

tryptophan   an amino acid that can be found in many animal proteins. It aids the body in production of niacin, which helps produce serotonin, a natural sedative.

vasoconstriction   the process in which blood vessels constrict to limit the blood flow to a particular area of the body.

vasodilation   dilation of the blood vessels (especially the arteries) in order to allow more blood to flow to a particular area of

yo-yo dieting   eating pattern which consists of widely varying extremes, such as binging and purging.

Notes

Part One

!Kung San:
http://www.ucc.uconn.edu/~epsadm03/Kung.html, http://www.essortment.com/all/
kungsanpeople_rftw.htm, http://abbott-infotech.co.za/tribes%20in%20the%20kalahari.
html, http://www.beyondveg.com/tu-j-l/raw-cooked/raw-cooked-3f.shtml

What's on the menu

/Du/da hunter/gatherers: Lee (1999:155). Resettlement: http://www.iol.co.za/index.
php?sf=68&set_id=1&click_id=68&art_id=qw1157430961698B213, http://www.youtube.
com/watch?v=XU-PceRraU0 Hunter/gatherer health: Cordain (2000), O'Dea (1984). Raw
plant toxins: http://www.beyondveg.com/tu-j-l/raw-cooked/raw-cooked-1g.shtml, http://
www.nutrition4health.org/NOHAnews/NNF01SoyBeatrice.htm

The Evolution Diet

Goddess: http://cas.bellarmine.edu/tietjen/images/neolithic_agriculture.htm

The Purpose of a Diet

Yo-yo Dieting: http://www.med.umich.edu/opm/newspage/2003/yoyodiet.htm. Genes:
Britten (2004); http://news.nationalgeographic.com/news/2002/09/0924_020924_
dnachimp.html. Obesity: ttp://www.healthinsite.gov.au/content/internal/page.
cfm?ObjID=000333EF-EC5C-1E1C-940083032BFA006D. Fewer genes: http://txtwriter.
com/Onscience/Articles/fewgenes.html. How food works: http://home.howstuffworks.
com/food.htm

Part Two

Lartoli footprints: McKie (2000). Bipedalism and hunter/gatherer behavior: http://www.
pbs.org/wgbh/nova/allfours/bipe-nf.html

Digestive Tract

Eat Our Colors: http://chppm-www.apgea.army.mil/dhpw/Wellness/SavorSpectrum.
jpg. Health magazine, April 2004. Stomach acidity: http://www.smartskincare.com/
skinbiology/sebum.html. Decreased oral health: Larsen 1998. Scissor-like motion: Klein
(1999:204). Chimps: Harris (1989:37-38). Dogs are color blind: http://www.uwsp.edu/
psych/dog/LA/DrP4.htm. Stomach acidity: http://www.smartskincare.com/skinbiology/
sebum.html. Chivers quote: Chivers (1992: 64). Digestive system: http://digestive.niddk.nih.
gov/ddiseases/pubs/yrdd/index.htm. Animals' digestive tract: http://www.hillstrath.on.ca/
moffatt/bio3a/digestive/vartheme.htm

How A Dynamic Physiology Helps Humans

Peter Wheeler: McKie (2000: 23). Harris quote: Harris (1989:148).

Part Three

Fogel: Fogel (1999). French fries: http://www.rense.com/general7/whyy.htm

The Culture-less Diet

Neotame: http://www.neotame.com/about.asp. Disgusting Foods: D'Amato, Erik (1998).
African insect food: http://www.si.edu/resource/faq/nmnh/buginfo/inasfood.htm

What A Culture-less Person Would Eat

Sedentary lifestyle: Larsen, 1995; Fermentation: Rush (2000); Chivers (1994:60-64). Grains: Kushi (1993). Mastadons: http://www.unmuseum.org/missingm.htm. Vitamins: http://www.nwhealth.edu/healthyU/eatWell/vitamins_1.html, http://www.ext.colostate.edu/PUBS/foodnut/09312.html. Iroquois and Cracker Jacks: http://cuyahogafallshistory.com/Beginnings/native_american_food.htm, http://www.crackerjack.com/nutrition.php

Cultural Influences

Neophobia: Logue (2000: 90). Harris quotes: Harris (1989:168, 155).

Personal Influences

Erik D'Amato: http://psychologytoday.com/articles/pto-19980201-000032.html. Taste Aversion Learning: Logue, (2000: 93)

Part Four

Carbohydrate Is Not A Four Letter Word

Quote: http://www.yalemedicalgroup.org/news/ymg_archive.html. High Fiber: http://www.healthcastle.com/candiettx_08_02.shtml. MedStar Study: http://jama.ama-assn.org/cgi/content/full/295/1/39.

What Too Much Sugar Does To Us

Diabetes: http://diabetes.about.com/library/blnews/blnobesityenzyme1201.htm, http://my.webmd.com/hw/diabetes_1_2/uq1444.asp?lastselectedguid={5FE84E90-BC77-4056-A91C-9531713CA348}. Quote: Rush (2000). Islets of Langerhans: http://www.medterms.com/script/main/art.asp?articlekey=4054. Blood sugar: http://www.prosperityplace.com/bdy_mind/bldsgar.html. Snickers: http://www.mmmars.com/cai/snickers/faq.html

We Are Made of Protein

Protein: Harris (1989:306-7). Protein Metabolism: http://www.trans4mind.com/personal_development/nutrition/stress/BodyStress.htm, http://insulin-pumpers.org/howto/pfandbs-2.html. More energy with high-carb diet: Truth About Food: Find Out If a High-Carb Diet Really Gives People More Energy (Video: 2007). Protein digestion: Strader, et al. (2005:175-191), http://www.womentowomen.com/digestionandgihealth/phbalance.asp, http://en.wikipedia.org/wiki/Digestion#Stomach. Digestion diseases: Adams (1999). Tryptophan: http://recipes.howstuffworks.com/question519.htm

With Friends Like Fats, Who Needs Enemies

Cholesterol: http://www.americanheart.org/presenter.jhtml?identifier=180. Fatty acid ratio: http://www.webmd.com/diet/guide/good-fat-bad-fat-facts-about-omega-3. Omega-3: http://www.biodynamics.net.au/articles/omega_3/Omega%203%20Fatty%20Acids.doc. Trans-fats: http://www.fda.gov/fdac/features/2003/503_fats.html.

Part Five

Food allergies: http://en.wikipedia.org/wiki/Food_allergies. Pine nuts: http://www.faiusa.org/?page=treenuts. Deaths: Alasalvar (2008:65). Anaphylaxis description: http://www.foodallergy.org/anaphylaxis/index.html.

Dairy

History: Tannahill (1995:24-5). Milk and Chinese: http://www.card.iastate.edu/iowa_ag_

review/summer_04/article5.aspx, Harris (1989:167). Life expectancy: http://geography.
about.com/library/weekly/aa042000b.htm.

Egg

History: http://www.foodtimeline.org/foodeggs.html. Salmonella: http://
www.wrongdiagnosis.com/s/salmonella_food_poisoning/prevalence.htm.
Cholesterol: http://yourtotalhealth.ivillage.com/cholesterol, http://www.
calorieking.com/foods/calories-in-eggs-chicken-egg-egg-white-cooked-
no-added-fat_f-Y2lkPTE2MDcxJmJpZD0xJmZpZD05OTE1NSZlaWQ9NDlyN
Tg0MDU4JnBvcz0xJnBhcj0ma2V5PWVnZyB3aGl0ZQ.html. Egg allergy: http://en.wikipedia.
org/wiki/Egg_allergy.

Peanut

Bertolomé de las Casas: Smith (2000: 2).Diffusion: http://lanra.anthro.uga.edu/peanut/
knowledgebase/#intro."Mediocre taste": Smith (2000: 3). Lectins: Freed (1999:1023),
http://www.krispin.com/lectin.html, http://www.independent.co.uk/life-style/health-and-
wellbeing/health-news/eat-your-greens--but-easy-on-the-peanuts-726527.html, http://
www.myctm.org/articles/JF-blood-type-diet.php.

Seafood

Allergy: http://foodallergies.about.com/od/seafoodallergies/p/fishallergy.htm. Prehistoric
fish eating: http://www.fao.org/DOCREP/003/V8490E/V8490E03.htm. FAAN study: http://
www.consumerreports.org/cro/health-fitness/diseases-conditions/seafood-allergies-605/
overview/.

Shellfish

Allergy: http://foodallergies.about.com/od/seafoodallergies/p/shellfish.htm. Szabo quote:
http://www.manandmollusc.net/history_food.html. 2 percent of adults: Wood (2007:56).

Soy

History, Navarette quote: http://www.nsrl.uiuc.edu/aboutsoy/history1.html, http://
findarticles.com/p/articles/mi_hb6404/is_n2_v55/ai_n28640638/. Prevalence: http://www.
thesoyfoodscouncil.com/soyproteinallergy.html. Toxins: http://www.soyonlineservice.
co.nz/03toxins.htm. Protese inhibitors: http://www.foodrevolution.org/what_about_soy.
htm. Phytic acid: http://www.rebuild-from-depression.com/blog/2007/12/soy_and_
phytic_acid_stick_with.html, Tait (1983:75). Soyatoxin: Becker-Ritt (2004), http://www.ufrgs.
br/laprotox/cntx-urease-eng.htm. Nitrosamines: Haas (2006:474), http://www.ncbi.nlm.
nih.gov/pubmed/10797279. Denatured soy products: http://www.rwood.com/Articles/
Soy_Toxin_or_Tonic.htm.

Tree nuts

Almond: http://en.wikipedia.org/wiki/Almond. Tree nuts: Alasalvar (2008:65). Cashews:
http://www.wisegeek.com/are-raw-cashews-really-poisonous.htm. Brazil nuts: http://
waynesword.palomar.edu/ecoph1.htm. Cashews: http://www.wisegeek.com/are-raw-
cashews-really-poisonous.htm. Walnut: http://trees.suite101.com/article.cfm/the_black_
walnut_tree. Prevalence: Alasalvar (2008:68). Monounsaturated fat: http://www.annecollins.
com/dietary-fat/monounsaturated.htm.

Wheat

History and Andrews quote: http://www.foodtimeline.org/foodfaq2.html#wheat.
Intolerance: http://www.foodintol.com/wheat.asp, http://en.wikipedia.org/wiki/Celiac_
disease. Phytates: http://www.ncbi.nlm.nih.gov/pubmed/2820048.

Enck quote: Enck (2007).

Part Six

Listen to Your Body

Penn State Study: http://www.usatoday.com/news/health/2007-10-23-apple-diet_N.htm

Appropriate Your Diet

Toxicity: http://www.anyvitamins.com/vitamin-c-ascorbicacid-info.htm. Thermic effect: http://www.caloriesperhour.com/tutorial_thermic.php

Avoid Intake of Artificially Extreme Foods

Caffeine: http://www.meinl.com/CoffeeService/quality/facts.htm; Field et. Al (2003), http://magma.nationalgeographic.com/ngm/0501/feature1/, J.J. Barone, H.R. Roberts (1996:119-129). Tortilla Chips: http://my.webmd.com/content/pages/7/3220_282. htm?printing=true#2. World Obesity: http://www.bbc.co.uk/apps/ifl/skillswise/ gigaquiz?path=inthenews/2003/0123&infile=0123&pool=numbers10. Caffeine content: http://www.cspinet.org/new/cafchart.htm

Part Eight

Truman Everts: Langford (1972: 1), http://www.ruhooked.com/artman/article_638.shtml, http://www.yellowstonepark.com/MoreToKnow/ShowNewsDetails.aspx?newsid=1. Lewis and Clark and the Nez Perce: http://www.pbs.org/lewisandclark/native/nez.html, Benson (1982: 15-20). Pilgrims: Berzok, Murray (2005: 19-20). Reduction of variety: http://www.idrc. ca/en/ev-31631-201-1-DO_TOPIC.html.

Live Off the Land

Acorn mush: http://www.cccoe.net/miwokproject/Lesson3.html , Edible plants: http:// www.the-ultralight-site.com/edible-plants.html, Army Survival Manual (1999: 9-9-11), http://www.botgard.ucla.edu/html/botanytextbooks/economicbotany/Saccharum/index. html, http://www.wisegeek.com/what-are-bamboo-shoots.htm, http://www.wilderness- survival.net/plants-1.php, http://www.uq.edu.au/_School_Science_Lessons/TaroProj.html, http://www.victoria-adventure.org/aquatic_plants/recipes/taro_basics.html, http://www. living-foods.com/articles/rawcashew.html, http://www.ibiblio.org/pfaf/cgi-bin/arr_html?A gave+utahensis+eborispina, http://en.wikipedia.org/wiki/Date_palm

'Tis the Season

French habits: Pettinger (2006). Four plants: http://www.nytimes.com/2007/01/28/ magazine/28nutritionism.t.html?pagewanted=all. Healthier meats: http://www. nutraingredients.com/news/ng.asp?id=34395-omega-from-meat. Seasonal Foods: http:// www.sysindia.com/kitchen/svegis.html, http://www.crisco.com/basics/seasonal/winter.asp

Part Nine

Water: Chan, Knutsen, Blix, Lee, Fraser American Journal of Epidemiology Vol. 155, No. 9: 827-833, http://www.highvibrations.org/archive3/water.htm. http://www.naturodoc. com/library/nutrition/water.htm. Percentages: http://waltonfeed.com/self/h2ocont. html. Plentiful: Harris (1989: 134). Aboriginal water: http://lowchensaustralia.com/names/ abornames.htm. Aborigines: Bayly (1999).

Part Ten

Fad Diets: http://www.faddiet.com/rusairfordie.html. Milk: http://www.askdrsears.com/ html/4/T040600.asp. Amygdalin: http://www.nslc.wustl.edu/courses/Bio343A/2005/wheat. pdf. Broccoli: http://www.vegparadise.com/highestperch44.html. Tuna: http://www.atuna. com/species/species_datasheets.htm . Chicken: http://www.foodtimeline.org/foodmeats.

html. Spinach: http://www.cliffordawright.com/history/spinach.html. Calcium: Miller (2000).

Part Eleven

Basal Metabolism

BMR: http://www.thedietchannel.com/weightloss3.htm. BMR and breathing: http://www.encyclopedia.com/html/m1/metabolism.asp

The Origin of Exercise

Male/female track and field: Harris (1989: 278). Carrier: Carrier (1984).

The Importance of Exercise

Exercise expenditure: http://www.netfit.co.uk/fatcal.htm.

Breathing and Sleep

Sleep Foods: Sears (2002).

Stress

Stress and Sleep: http://www.annecollins.com/weight-loss-support/stress-overweight.htm. Stress and weightloss: http://www.annecollins.com/weight-loss-support/stress-overweight.htm.

Part Twelve

Health care costs: http://www.consumeraffairs.com/news04/2006/09/healthcare_costs.html, http://www.cnn.com/2004/HEALTH/conditions/01/21/obesity.spending.ap/.

Bibliography

Abrams, H L. "The Preference for Animal Protein and Fat: a Cross-Cultural Survey." Food and Evolution: Toward a Theory of Human Food Habits. Philadelphia: Temple UP, 1987. 207-223.

Adams, P F., G E. Hendershot, and M A. Marano. Current Estimates From the National Health Interview Survey, 1996. National Center for Health Statistics. National Center for Health Statistics, 1999. 200.

Alasalvar, Cesarettin. Tree Nut Nutraceuticals and Phytochemicals (Nutraceutical Science and Tech). CRC, 2008.

Ardrey, Robert. African Genesis: a Personal Investigation Into the Animal Origins and Nature of Man. New York: Athenaeum, 1961.

Audette, Ray. NeanderThin: Eat Like a Caveman to Achieve a Lean, Strong, Healthy Body. St. Martin Paperbacks, 2000.

Barone, J J., and H R. Roberts. "Caffeine Consumption." Food Chemistry and Toxicology 34 (1996): 119-129.

Barzun, Jacques. From Dawn to Decadence. New York: HarperCollins, 2000.

Bateson, Patrick, David Barker, Timothy Clutton-Brock, Deb Debal, Bruno D'udine, Robert A. Foley, Peter Gluckman, Keith Godfrey, Tom Kirkwood, Marta M. Lahr, John

McNamara, Nell Metcalfe, Patricial Monaghan, Hamish G. Spencer, and Sonia E. Sultan. "Developmental Plasticity and Human Health." 430: 419-421.

Bayly, I A E. "Review of How Indigenous People Managed for Water in Desert Regions of Australia." Journal of the Royal Society of Western Australia 82 (1999): 17-25.

Beadle, G. "The Ancestor of Corn." Scientific American 242 (1981): 96-103.

Becker-Ritt, Arlete B., Fernanda Mulinari, Ilka M. Vasconcelos, and Célia R. Carlini. "Antinutritional and/or toxic factors in soybean (Glycine max (L) Merril) seeds: comparison of different cultivars adapted to the southern region of Brazil." Journal of the Science of Food and Agriculture 84 (2004): 263-70.

Benson, Ragnar. Live Off the Land in the City and Country. New York: Paladin P, 1982. 15-20.

Berzok, Linda M. American Indian Food (Food in American History). New York: Greenwood P, 2005.

Bohan, Michelle, Lloyd Anderson, Allen Trenkle, and Donald Beitz. Effects of Dietary Macronutrients on Appetite-Related Hormones in Blood on Body Composition of Lean and Obese Rats. Iowa State University. 2006. 1-6.

Bouchez, Collett. "Yo-Yo Dieting Tugs on Your Heart's Strings." Health Day. 05 June 2005 <http://www.healthday.com/view.cfm?id=511643>.

Bowen, R. "Ghrelin." Colorado State University. 3 Sept. 2006. Colorado State University. 27 Oct. 2007 <http://arbl.cvmbs.colostate.edu/hbooks/pathphys/endocrine/gi/ghrelin.html>.

Brain, C K. The Hunters or the Hunted. Chicago: University of Chicago P, 1981.

Britten, Roy J. DNA Sequence Insertion and Evolutionary Variation in Gene Regulation. Biology of Developmental Transcription Control, 26 Oct. 1995, National Academy of Sciences. 1996.

Brody, Jane E. "It's Not Just the Calories, It's Their Source." New York Times 12 July 1988, sec. C3.

Calbet, J A L., and D A. Maclean. "Role of Caloric Content on Gastric Emptying in Humans." Journal of Physiology 498 (1997): 553-559.

Carrier, David. "The Energetic Paradox of Human Running and Hominid Evolution." Current Anthropology 25 (1984): 483-495.

Chagnon, Napoleon, and R Hames. "Protein Deficiency and Tribal Warfare in Amazonia: New Data." Sience 203 (1979): 910-913. Abstract. Science.

Chan, Hacqueline, Synnove F. Krutsen, Glen G. Blix, Jerry W. Lee, and Gary E. Fraser. "Water, Other Fluids, and Fatal Coronary Heart Disease." American Journal of Epidemiology 155 (2002): 827-833.

Chivers, David J., and C M. Hladik. "Morphology of the Gastrointestinal Tract in Primates: Comparisons with Other Mammals in Relation to Diet." Journal of Morphology 166. Abstract. Journal of Morphology 166 (2005): 377-386.

Cichoke, Anthony J. The Complete Book of Enzyme Therapy. New York: Avery, 1998. 10-20.

Cohen, Mark. The Food Crisis in Prehistory. New Haven: Yale UP, 1977.

Cordain, Loren. The Paleo Diet: Lose Weight and Get Healthy by Eating the Food You Were Designed to Eat. New York: Wiley, 2002.

Cordain, Loren, Janette Miller, S. Eaton, Neil Mann, Susanne Holt, and John Speth. "Plant-animal subsistence ratios and macronutrient energy estimations in worldwide hunter-gatherer diets." Am. J. Clinical Nutrition 71 (2000): 682-92.

D'amato, Erik. "The Mystery of Disgust - Reflections on What Disgusts People." Psychology

Today (1998).

"Digestive Diseases Statistics." National Digestive Diseases Information Clearinghouse. Dec. 2005. National Institiute of Diabetes and Digestive and Kidney Diseases. 12 Oct. 2007 <http://digestive.niddk.nih.gov/statistics/statistics.htm>.

Diliberti, Nicole, Peter L. Bordi, Martha T. Conklin, Liane S. Roe, and Barbara J. Rolls. "Increased Portion Size Leads to Increased Energy Intake in a Restaurant Meal." Obesity Research 12 (2004): 562-568.

Draper, Patricia, and Nancy Howell. Nutritional Status of !Kung Children. Conference on Hunting and Gathering Societies, Edinburgh, Scotland, 2002. 2002.

Dufour, Dama. "Insects as Food: a Case Study From the Northwest Amazon." American Anthropologist 89 (1986): 383-397.

Eldredge, Niles, and Ian Tattersall. The Myths of Human Evolution. New York: Columbia UP, 1982.

Enck, Paul. "Psychological burden of food allergy." World Journal of Gastroenterology 13 (2007): 3456-465.

Field, Aaron S., Paul J. Laurienti, Yi-Fen Yen, Johnathan H. Burdette, and Dixon M. Moody. "Dietary Caffeine Consumption and Withdrawal: Confounding Variables in Quantitative Cerebral Perfusion Studies." Radiology (2003): 129-135. Abstract. Radiology (2003).

Fogel, Robert W. United States. Food and Rural Economics Division. US Department of Agriculture. America's Eating Habits: Changes and Consequences. Washington, D.C., 1999.

Fritz, Gayle. "New Dates and Data on Early Agriculture: the Legacy of Complex Hunter-Gatherers." Annals of the Missouri Botanical Garden 82 (1995): 3-15.

Goodman, Alan H., R B. Thomas, A C. Swedlund, and G Armelagos. "Biocultural Perspectives on Stress in Prehistoric, Historical, and Contemporary Population Research." American Journal of Physical Anthropology 31 (1988): 169-202. Abstract. InterScience (2005).

Goscienski, Philip J. Health Secrets of the Stone Age, Second Edition. Oceanside, CA: Better Life, 2005.

Gunnell, D., S. E. Oliver, T. J. Peters, J. L. Donovan, R. Persad, M. Maynard, D. Gillatt, A. Pearce, F. C. Hamdy, D. E. Neal, and J. M P Holly. "Are diet?prostate cancer associations mediated by the IGF axis? A cross-sectional analysis of diet, IGF-1 and IGFBP-3 in healthy middle-aged men." British Journal of Cancer 88 (2003): 1682-686.

Haas, Elson M., and Buck Levin. Staying Healthy With Nutrition, 21st Century Edition The Complete Guide to Diet & Nutritional Medicine. New York: Celestial Arts, 2006.

Hansen, J D L. "Hunter-Gatherer to Pastoral Way of Life: Effects of the Transition on Health, Growth, and Nutritional Status." Southern African Journal of Science 89 (1993): 559-567.

Harris, Marvin. Good to Eat: Riddles of Food and Culture. New York: Simon and Schuster, 1985.

Harris, Marvin. Our Kind. New York: Harper & Row, 1989.

Hiraiwa, M, R W. Byrne, H Takasaki, and J M. Byrne. "Aggression Toward Large Carnivores by Wild Chimpanzees of Mahale Mountains Nation Park, Tanzania." Folia Primatol (Basel) 47 (1986): 8-13. Abstract. PubMed.

Iggulden, Conn, and Hal Iggulden. The Dangerous Book for Boys. New York: HarperCollins,

2006.

Jenike, M R. "Seasonal Hunger Among Tropical Africans: the Lese Case." American Journal of Physical Anthropology 78 (1989): 247.

Klein, R. The Human Career: Human Biological and Cultural Origins, 2nd Edition. Chicago: University of Chicago P, 1999.

Lee, Richard B., and Irven Devore. Kalahari Hunter-Gatherers Studies of the !Kung San & Their Neighbors. Lincoln: IUniverse, 1999.

Lewin, Roger. "Man the Scavenger." Science 224 (1984): 861-862.

Logue, Alexandra. The Psychology of Eating and Drinking. New York: Brunner-Routledge, 2004.

McKie, Robin. Dawn of Man: the Story of Human Evolution. London: BBC Worldwide Ltd., 2000.

Mela, D.j. "Food Choice and Intake: the Human Factor." Proceedings of the Nutrition Society Volume 58, Number 3 (1999): 513-521. Abstract. Ingentaconnect.

Mercola, Joseph. Dr. Mercola's Total Health Program: the Proven Plan to Prevent Disease and Premature Aging, Optimize Weight and Live Longer. Schaumburg, IL: Mercola.Com, 2003.

Miller, Gregory D. "Year 2000 Dietary Guidelines: New Thoughts for a New Millennium." American Society for Clinical Nutrition 71 (2000): 657-664.

Morwood, Mike, Thomas Sutikna, and Richard Roberts. "The People Time Forgot." National Geographic Apr. 2005: 2.

Nishida, Toshisada. "The Ant-Gathering Behavior by the Use of Tools Among Wild Chimpanzees of the Mahale Mountains." Journal of Human Evolution 2 (1973): 357-370.

O'Dea, K. "Marked improvement in carbohydrate and lipid metabolism in diabetic Australian aborigines after temporary reversion to traditional lifestyle." Diabetes 33 (1984): 596-603.

Oz, Mehmet C., and Michael F. Roizen. You: on a Diet: the Owner's Manual for Waist Management. New York: Free P, 2006.

Pettinger, Claire, Michelle Holdsworth, and Mariette Gerber. "Meal Patterns and Cooking Practices in Southern France and Central England." Public Health Nutrition 9 (2006): 1020-1026. Abstract. Public Health Nutrition.

Pollan, Michael. The Omnivore's Dilemma: a Natural History of Four Meals. New York: Penguin P HC, 2006.

Price, Douglas, and James Brown. Prehistoric Hunter-Gatherers: the Emergence of Cultural Complexity. New York: Academic P, 1985.

Pusztai, A. Plant lectins. Cambridge: Cambridge UP, 1991.

Reid, T R. "Caffeine." National Geographic Jan. 2005: 2-33.

Ridley, Matt. Nature Via Nurture. New York: HarperCollins, 2003.

Rush, John A. "Applying Medical Anthropology: Gut Morphology, Cultural Eating Habits, Digestive Failure, and Ill Health." MedAnth. 7 Aug. 2005 <http://www.medanth.org/case_studies/rush01.htm>.

Ruskin, Jeremy. "The Fast Food Trap: How Commercialism Creates Overweight Children - Special Report: Kids and Corporate Culture." Mothering Nov.-Dec. 2003.

Shipman, Pat. "Scavenging or Hunting in Early Hominids: Theoretical Framework and Tests." American Anthropologist 88 (1986): 27-43. Abstract. JSTOR.

Smith, Andrew F. Peanuts the illustrious history of the goober pea. Urbana: University of Illinois P, 2002.

Strader, April D., and Stephen D. Woods. "Gastrointestinal Hormones and Food Intake." Abstract. Gastroenterology 131 (2005): 175-191.

"Stress: Treatment." National Women's Health Resource Centers. 1 May 2005 <http://health.ivillage.com/mindbody/mbstress/0,,nwhrc_75hm0msw,00.html?iv_arrivalSA=1&iv_cobrandRef=0&iv_arrival_freq=1&pba=adid=16657989>.

Tait, S. "The availability of minerals in food, with particular reference to iron." Journal of Research in Society & Health 103 (1983): 74-77.

Tannahill, Reay. Food in History. New York: Three Rivers P, 1995.

Truth About Food: Find Out If a High-Carb Diet Really Gives People More Energy. Mehmet Oz. Discovery Health. 25 Sept. 2007 <http://health.discovery.com/convergence/truth/video.html>.

"Typical Caloric Density Information." Dyets. 10 Aug. 2005 <http://www.dyets.com/caloric.htm>.

United States. The National Cancer Institute's. The National Cancer Institute's (NCI) 5 a Day for Better Health Program. Washington, D.C., 1999.

United States. U.S. Department of Health and Human Services and U.S. Department of Agriculture. Dietary Guidelines for Americans, 2005. Washington, D.C.: U.S. Government Printing Office, 2005.

United States Department Of Defense. US Army Survival Manual: FM 21-76. Washington, D.C.: Department of the Army, 1970.

Warner, Jennifer. "Skinny Smokers Just as Unhealthy." Web MD. 27 Oct. 2005 <http://my.webmd.com/content/article/24/1837_50611.htm>.

Waterlow, J C. "Metabolic Adaptation to Low Intakes of Energy and Protein." Annual Review of Nutrition 6 (1986): 495-520.

Wood, Robert, and Joe Kraynak. Food Allergies For Dummies. New york: For Dummies, 2007.

LaVergne, TN USA
14 July 2010
189500LV00004B/177/P